FATAL CARE

SURVIVE
IN THE U.S.
HEALTH SYSTEM

BY SANJAYA
KUMAR, MD

FOREWORD BY
DAVID B. NASH, MD

IGI PRESS . MINNEAPOLIS

Photo Acknowledgments
All photos are from the collections of the families in each story except for the image of
Thursday Jeffers on page 233, which is courtesy of WRTV 6 News, Indianapolis, IN.

Visit the book's Web site: www.fatalcare.com

Published by IGI PRESS
241 First Ave. No.
Minneapolis, MN 55401

Library of Congress Cataloging-in-Publication Data

Kumar, Sanjaya, 1963–
  Fatal care : survive in the U.S. health system / by Sanjaya Kumar.
     p. cm.
  ISBN 978-0-9777121-1-3
  1. Medical errors—United States. 2. Medical care—United States. I. Title.
  R729.8.K86 2008
  610—dc22

                                  2008003141

Manufactured in the United Stated of America (USA)
6 5 4 3 2 1 – BP – 13 12 11 10 09 08

AUTHOR'S NOTE

This book is narrative nonfiction with dramatization of fatal or
potentially serious preventable medical errors and adverse events
that have occurred in the recent past. The characters portrayed in
the stories are real and the events described are based on factual
information, told to the best of my understanding from research
conducted. Where necessary, names have been changed to provide
privacy and anonymity for those involved. Passages in which I narrate
a person's thoughts and feelings and present dialogue have been built
from interviews with the subjects, witnesses, and those involved, and
have been fact-checked for correctness of information included.

There are an untold number of fatal, preventable medical errors
occurring everyday. Many go unrecognized, with only a few garnering
the attention they deserve. It is from these stories that we can learn
to be less afraid and empower ourselves to be safer. So many stories
never get told. My goal is to reveal the underlying systems issues, the
people involved, their lives, and the impact of such errors on those
involved and us as future patients.

Sanjaya Kumar, M.D.
February 14, 2008

DISCLAIMER

The cases and stories in this book are true. The real names of victims and their family members have been used, however the names of physicians, healthcare professionals and hospital facilities have either been omitted or changed to fictional names; and in some cases, the person's gender has been changed. The fictional names of physicians and care givers used are not to represent any other real physician or care giver with the same or similar name. This has been done because *Fatal Care* purposely tells the story from the "patient's eyes" and provides a platform for their experience. It is about the patient and their perspective, it is about their story.

While every effort has been made to ensure the accuracy of the information and material contained in this book, the author, publisher and all others associated with the research, production, distribution, marketing and sales of the book or related materials assume no responsibility for the accuracy or completeness of the information provided, and they accept no liability. The information and examples contained in this book are not intended as a substitute for professional medical advice. Please contact your physician for any concerns or questions about medical care.

FOR MY FATHER

Mahesh Chandra

*A man of principles; I would not be
who I am without his encouragement,
guidance and integrity*

AND

*For the patients who became victims
of the healthcare system they trusted
to make them better*

"*I swear by Apollo, Asclepius, Hygieia, and Panacea, and I take to witness all the gods, all the goddesses, to keep according to my ability and my judgment, the following Oath.*

To consider dear to me, as my parents, him who taught me this art; to live in common with him and, if necessary, to share my goods with him; To look upon his children as my own brothers, to teach them this art.

I will prescribe regimens for the good of my patients according to my ability and my judgment and never do harm to anyone.

To please no one will I prescribe a deadly drug nor give advice which may cause his death.

Nor will I give a woman a pessary to procure abortion.

But I will preserve the purity of my life and my arts.

I will not cut for stone, even for patients in whom the disease is manifest; I will leave this operation to be performed by practitioners, specialists in this art.

In every house where I come I will enter only for the good of my patients, keeping myself far from all intentional ill-doing and all seduction and especially from the pleasures of love with women or with men, be they free or slaves.

All that may come to my knowledge in the exercise of my profession or in daily commerce with men, which ought not to be spread abroad, I will keep secret and will never reveal.

If I keep this oath faithfully, may I enjoy my life and practice my art, respected by all men and in all times; but if I swerve from it or violate it, may the reverse be my lot."

—The Hippocratic Oath, by Hippocrates
(translated from Greek), the Father of Medicine,
4th Century BC

(Source: Wikipedia, the free encyclopedia)

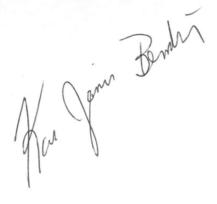

ACKNOWLEDGMENT

Writing this book has been a very special project for me, and a touching experience in many ways. I wish to express my heartfelt thanks to all those who were open and kind enough to share their painful (and in some cases tragic) stories for this literary work to get done. I was very much impressed with the willingness of those involved in medical errors to share their experience with others in the hopes of averting like mishaps, and a strong desire on their part to see that others not have to endure the agony they and their families had experienced. These are ordinary people, like you and me, with an enormous amount of compassion for humanity.

There were numerous people who helped shape the tenor of this book. My sincere thanks go to Karin Janine Berntsen, a colleague and author, for her tireless research into each of the stories and for guiding the construct of the stories covered in *Fatal Care*. Karin Berntsen is a contributory writer and researcher for the book *Fatal Care*. Her contribution and attention to the clinical and factual details of each story was invaluable. Ms. Berntsen is currently the President of PreventingMedicalErrors.com, a patient safety consultation company. Ms. Berntsen is an author, healthcare executive, registered nurse and certified patient safety officer with more than 25 years of healthcare experience. Her roles have included Vice President of Patient Safety, Chief Nursing Officer and Director of Risk Management, and Quality. Ms. Berntsen authored the book, *The Patient's Guide to Preventing Medical Errors* - Praeger Publishing Group, Westport, Connecticut.

I also wish to thank Pat Irwin for making these stories spring to life. From the beginning, the idea was to present the stories covered as "drama" in order to grip the reader into the lives of those involved and affected by the medical errors. Pat made this possible by patiently listening to Karin and me, and translating our concepts into unfolding dramatization of facts. Many thanks go to Chris Bethell who was an early advocate of this project and helped create a framework for each chapter and the work as a whole. I would also like to extend my deep appreciation to T.J. Tedesco for convincing me to start this project, and his literary direction and constant vigilance in keeping me on track with my timelines.

Thank you to the fine people at IGI Publishing, including Sue Corns, Gary Hansen and Zach Marell. This is a better book because of their diligent efforts.

Last, but not the least, I would like to thank my dear wife (Sandy), my daughter (Sherie), and my two boys (Nishant and Manish) for their support and tolerance while I spent countless nights and weekends pouring over rewrites and edits of the manuscript. Without their willingness to share their husband and father during this period I would not have been able to write this book. I would also like to express my appreciation to my dear father and mother for their continued support of any and all of my professional and personal endeavors. Their guidance and direction has helped shape my path and for that I am forever grateful.

Finally, there are countless others who have influenced my life and indirectly made this book a reality. To these many untold friends and colleagues I offer my sincere thanks for their friendship and support.

FOREWORD

Nearly a decade ago, the Institute of Medicine's (IOM) Report on "To Err is Human" highlighted a major national epidemic of fatal medical errors within our healthcare system. In subsequent years following the IOM findings, the healthcare industry went through the various stages of denial, understanding and finally acceptance. During our industry's journey through these stages, the public has had a glimpse of the underlying structural and systemic defects in healthcare, and names like Betsy Lehman and Josie King have become a part of the national lexicon.

Yet, at the operational level, from hospitals to the primary care office, much more needs to be done to limit the incidence of preventable medical errors. Imagine the dreadful scenario of a fully loaded Boeing 747 airplane crashing and killing all aboard every day for a year at an American airport. After the first day of this grisly scenario, the FAA would shut down every plane and a dramatic nationwide self-evaluation of the entire aviation industry would occur. Every nut and bolt of every 747 worldwide would be inspected for visible and potential defects. Healthcare has no comparable ability to self-evaluate, repair and move on. Enter, Dr. Sanjaya Kumar and his wonderful new book *Fatal Care*.

Fatal Care gives a face and a name to every passenger on those fictitious crashing airplanes. *Fatal Care* links a decade's worth of work about what's wrong with our system to a fresh look at possible solutions for the unsuspecting "victim," who is potentially you and me. Finally, *Fatal Care* presents the entire package in a readable, compassionate and gripping manner. This book is a virtual "how to guide" for all of the key stakeholders in that it will help to redefine professionalism. Sanjaya Kumar will help medicine recognize that professionalism really means a willingness to self-evaluate and improve performance based on real data and introspection grounded in reality. It means we have to take apart every nut and bolt, inspect it, improve it, and put the entire system back together again.

These are not all happy stories with happy endings. *Fatal Care* is composed of real stories filled with high drama, pathos and unforgettable individual characters. Sanjaya Kumar maintains a focus on powerful cultural barriers resistant to changes within our healthcare system. As repeatedly shown, today's healthcare systems are rife with cultures devoted to autonomous decision-making despite clear evidence of unsafe practices, preventable deaths and destruction. *Fatal Care* provides a hope for the future with specific suggestions for improvement backed by real world information for today's all too real healthcare consumers.

Sanjaya Kumar and his colleagues at Quantros are leading the way toward the future as we collectively build a safer healthcare system, albeit too slowly for his tastes and mine. We need every patient, every doctor and every hospital leader to read *Fatal Care* as a guidebook toward a practical vision of a much safer future. Our patients, families and generations-to-come deserve no less. Kudos to Dr. Sanjaya Kumar for leading the way.

David B. Nash, MD, MBA
Professor and Chairman
Department of Health Policy
Jefferson Medical College
Philadelphia, Pennsylvania

Contents

PROLOGUE

Today, if you are in the market for a particular type of car you can easily use the expansive reaches of the Internet to research features, performance, safety, and quality information on hundreds of vehicles without leaving the comfort of your home. You can visit countless websites where you can find the most recent safety ratings, crash test figures, rollover test ratings and detailed specifications on each make and model. You can even compare selected models side by side, allowing you to make an informed decision on what you want to invest in based on feature sets, options, safety rankings, durability, and retail price. As knowledge rich and empowered "consumers" the choice is yours to make on what kind of wheels you buy. You can pay less and buy a cheaper car that might not necessarily be the safest or spend more and buy a car that has a five star crash rating. Overall the goal of these sophisticated data and information rich sites is to offer potential customers the opportunity to make an informed decision that may one day save their lives.

Now consider what is available to you when you're looking for a new physician for routine care, or when you need a procedure that requires a hospital stay. Often, you first turn to friends or coworkers for word-of-mouth references. But if you are seeking the same kind of useful patient safety data on your local area physicians and hospitals that you can obtain about cars, you're out of luck. Nowhere can healthcare consumers find transparent information on the

6-11

THE NUMBER OF PREVENTABLE DEATHS EVERY HOUR IN U.S. HOSPITALS AS A RESULT OF MEDICAL MISTAKES

Source: Kohn, L.T, Corrigan, J.M. & Donaldson, M.S. (Eds.). (1999). To err is human: building a safer health system. Institute of Medicine. Washington, D.C.: National Academy Press.

patient safety records of healthcare providers and institutions, despite the fact that your life and health may hang in the balance. In spite of the "knowledge boom" for something as basic to life as healthcare services there are few, if any, comprehensive places on the Internet to shop and compare for what we might need from the healthcare industry.

The lack of information is truly ironic when you consider that, annually, as many as 98,000 patient deaths are estimated to occur in the U.S. as a result of medical errors in hospitals and more than half are preventable. This is equivalent to losing one commercial jumbo jet airliner full of about 270 passengers each day, every day of the year or about 11 preventable fatalities every hour of any given day. As devastating as any epidemic, preventable medical errors lead to more deaths than those from breast cancer, HIV/AIDS and traffic accidents combined. Medication errors alone are estimated to injure at least 1.5 million Americans annually, plus they add to the healthcare costs by about $3.5 billion.

Have you ever wondered why we have so many campaigns to fight against breast cancer or AIDS/HIV or DUI, but hardly any for

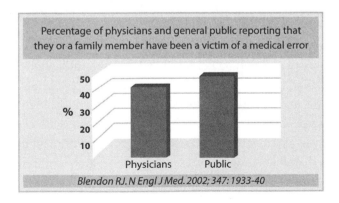

Percentage of physicians and general public reporting that they or a family member have been a victim of a medical error

Blendon RJ. N Engl J Med. 2002; 347: 1933-40

fighting preventable medical errors? Is this because we are too afraid to admit the truth—that one day we can be a victim? Or are we afraid, like a cancer victim, to learn the shocking reality of a fractured system that is in place to cater to our health and well-being?

Unfortunately, this silent epidemic doesn't receive the same attention an airline crash attracts. It's not as public and sensational, except for a few cases every now and then that come to surface, in many cases when someone famous is involved. In reality, this epidemic is far more devastating in sheer numbers of resulting deaths and the radiating impact on those affected by this "epidemic." You are never more vulnerable than when you place your life and well-being in the hands of healthcare professionals and the complex systems of care delivery that exist today. Each day, weak links in the healthcare system produce the majority of medical errors and compromise patient safety and the lives of patients.

As a patient in a hospital, you entrust your safety to others the moment you check in, assuming there are multiple processes in place to safeguard against preventable medical errors. You may believe your hospital and physician take every available precaution to create a system of checks and balances. Maybe you think serious, life-threatening mistakes could never happen to you or your loved ones. But you would be wrong, dead wrong.

Medical errors can happen to anyone, and at any institution. Shortly before this manuscript was sent to our publisher, the actor Dennis Quaid, his wife Kimberly Buffington and their family became a victim of a medical error when their infant twins were given a thousand times stronger dose of heparin than required. As you will soon discover, this episode has an eerily familiar feel to the events described in chapter eleven, which happened in an Indiana hospital fourteen months earlier.

It does not matter how big or small your checking account is, or to what part of society you belong. Well-known public figures and celebrities like the Quaids are not immune to the problem. Grave mistakes occur in small-town hospitals, as well as at some of the most prestigious medical facilities in the nation, and with alarming frequency. In the majority of cases these errors go unrecognized and unreported, and in some cases, are even deliberately covered up to avoid litigation.

People continue to trust a fractured health system when they seek treatment, unaware of the safety gaps and unintended risks. The current medical error rate demands that we take action as consumers. The healthcare industry needs to provide the same level of safety statistics, data and transparency that is found in other industries such as auto manufacturing or commercial aviation, where lives are on the line. Patients want and need to receive safe healthcare each and every time they seek treatment. In addition, healthcare professionals desire systems that will help them avoid mistakes. Through technology and improved systems, enormous progress can be made going forward.

A MESSAGE AND A MISSION

Fatal Care will take you on a journey, and introduce you to individuals and families living within the nameless, faceless world of medical error statistics. They are people like you and your relatives, your children, neighbors and friends, and their stories are as varied as their lives. Each one is unique and holds the drama, suspense and emotion that are part of life and death. But most importantly, each story has something to teach patients and healthcare professionals about how to avoid the pitfalls, or fatal points, along the course of care.

The stories included in this book are but a miniscule sampling of the thousands of other like cases. Each is based on actual events that have involved individuals like you, and has been carefully selected to depict an unknown and harrowing journey that leaves behind a trail of torment for all those that unexpectedly venture into its path. The stories portray and reveal the lives of those affected before and after the medical error, the inner workings of our "trusted" healthcare system, the introspective journey of the patient or family member in a thriller–like fashion, and the life altering aftermath.

The structures of the current health system shroud the truth about the extent of such unintended adverse events, suffered at the hands of trusted healthcare providers and hospitals. Many of us are simply too afraid to admit that tomorrow, we could be the next victims behind these statistics. Turning away out of fear of the unknown will not protect you; knowing how and why such things happen can better prepare you, and perhaps save your life or the life of a loved one in the future. *Fatal Care* provides a window into the lives of those affected and gives you, as a patient, the insights to avoid becoming the next casualty.

PATIENT SAFETY KNOWLEDGE SHARE

Preventable deaths — two major published peer reviewed studies reported that between 2.9% and 3.7% of all hospitalized patients experience an adverse event (AE), with 6.6%-13.6% of them followed by death. The Institute of Medicine's (IOM) well-known statistic of 44,000-98,000 deaths per year comes from using these two estimates (6.6% and 13.6%), projected over the roughly 30 million hospitalizations in the United States each year.

A more recent study specifically assessed the preventability of deaths among hospitalized patients. This study found that multiple reviewers judged 6% of hospital deaths as probably or definitely preventable. Using this result produces estimates of 115 and 302 death per million "opportunities" (annual hospital admissions in US),

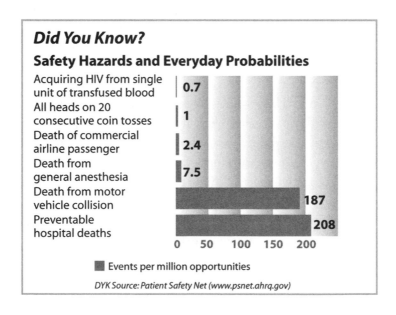

Did You Know?

Safety Hazards and Everyday Probabilities

	Events per million opportunities
Acquiring HIV from single unit of transfused blood	0.7
All heads on 20 consecutive coin tosses	1
Death of commercial airline passenger	2.4
Death from general anesthesia	7.5
Death from motor vehicle collision	187
Preventable hospital deaths	208

0   50   100   150   200

■ Events per million opportunities

DYK Source: Patient Safety Net (www.psnet.ahrq.gov)

depending on whether one chooses upper or lower bounds of the ranges for the adverse event rate (2.9%-3.7%) and the proportion of adverse events followed by death (6.6%-13.6 %). The figure shows 208 deaths per million, the average of these upper and lower bounds.

$17-29 Billion

ESTIMATED ANNUAL
COST OF PREVENTABLE
MEDICAL ERRORS
TO THE AMERICAN
ECONOMY (IN THE
FORM OF ADDITIONAL
HEALTHCARE COSTS,
LOST INCOME
AND HOUSEHOLD
PRODUCTION, AND
DISABILITY)

67%

PERCENTAGE OF
MEDICAL MISTAKES
OCCURRING IN
HOSPITALS THAT
COULD BE PREVENTED

Source: Hayward RA, Hofer TP. Estimating hospital deaths due to medical errors: preventability is in the eye of the reviewer. JAMA. 2001;286:415-420.

CHAPTER 1

NEVER ROUTINE

In this chapter

You will better understand why it is important to know the different titles and positions that physicians hold in hospitals, and what role each one plays.

- Learn when and how to go up the hospital chain of command when you have concerns about the care being provided or condition of a patient.
- Understand what is *failure to rescue*, and why it can be deadly?
- Find out about Rapid Response Teams (RRT) and why you need to know if your hospital has one.

*Why is "**failure to rescue**" important for you to know?*

Being cared for in the hospital is no guarantee of immediate intervention, should your condition rapidly deteriorate or if you develop a life-threatening complication. In a busy and sometimes understaffed hospital, serious, unexpected developments can go unchecked and warning signs and symptoms can be ignored or missed. In these circumstances, getting doctors and nurses to recognize the situation and act quickly can be the difference between life and death for you or your loved one.

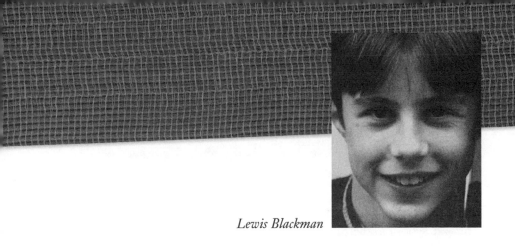

Lewis Blackman

Helen Haskell, a soft-spoken Southern woman, still has trouble comprehending what happened to her son, Lewis, when she relives the sequence of events that changed her world. When he entered the hospital for routine surgery on the morning of Thursday, November 2, 2000, Lewis Blackman was a healthy, active teenage boy, a model of youth and vigor brimming with potential. By the afternoon of Monday, November 6, he was lying in a hospital morgue, just blocks from the motel where his stunned family stayed as they awaited his autopsy results.

Only a month beyond his fifteenth birthday, Lewis Blackman was sampling his first taste of independence and was poised to do great things. With two months of high school under his belt and a brand new learner's permit (his most prized possession) in his wallet, a life of promise and unlimited possibilities was beginning to unfold.

Lewis had grown up in a home where education and learning were treasured commodities. When Lewis was born, his mother, Helen, was pursuing a graduate degree in archaeology. His father, Bar, was a teacher. After Lewis' sister Eliza was born five years later, Helen put her Ph.D. on hold and stayed home full-time with the children. They became her lifework. Helen taught Lewis what she knew, and taught him to love the things she loved.

As a young child, Lewis and his mother read from an atlas at bedtime, and she encouraged him to dream about the places he would go someday. He excelled in school, viewing subjects like physics and history as a form of recreation, and his natural curiosity spurred him to develop a broad knowledge about the world. Occasionally he acted in commercials and a local Shakespeare company.

Fortunately for Lewis, his personality and sense of humor protected him from being labeled a nerd by his peers. He managed to achieve that elusive balance between intelligence and popularity that few teenagers are able to pull off. Kind and empathetic, he was the first one to welcome a new student or befriend the kid others picked on. People liked Lewis and sought out his company.

The fall of 2000 was a hectic time of change for Lewis and his family. Lewis started his first year of high school at Hammond, a private school in their hometown of Columbia, S.C., where his parents hoped he would feel challenged. Eliza, now ten-years-old, took on as many activities as her brother. Helen had resumed working toward her Ph.D., and also began a campaign to make sure her children didn't go out into the world helpless. She implemented a regimen to teach Lewis and Eliza domestic skills like cooking and laundry, after discovering they knew even less about household chores than she had suspected. After all, in a few short years they would be launching Lewis into young adulthood when he went to college, and he would need to survive on his own.

College was looming on the horizon, a fact brought home to Helen and Bar when they took the kids on a trip to visit Duke University, their alma mater, on the last weekend in October of that year. Lewis loved the campus, and despite Duke's high admissions standards, his preliminary college-board exams, the highest in the Columbia area, suggested he would have little trouble getting into the school. His future looked brilliant.

That fall also became a convenient time to deal with a health issue Lewis had all his life, while he was still at home and in high school. Lewis was born with a congenital deformity called *pectus excavatum*, found in up to one in 400 people. Commonly known as *funnel chest* or *cobbler's chest*, those with the condition have a malformed, depressed sternum that causes the chest to have a concave, sunken appearance. Typically the depression of the breastbone deepens during adolescence when a child's bones grow most quickly, creating a bowl-shape. "You could eat cereal and milk out of my chest," Lewis quipped to his friends.

Over the years, Helen and Bar considered surgical correction for Lewis' defect, but the standard operation seemed so invasive and risky.

It could take up to five hours and required doctors to open the entire chest, removing ribs and cartilage. The recovery could be difficult and lengthy. Then in 1999 they read an article in the newspaper about a new, less invasive approach to correct pectus excavatum. The Nuss procedure, as it was called, required only two small incisions to insert a bar that slowly corrects the shape of the sternum over time. The entire procedure could be done in an hour. After two years, the bar would be removed during another simple surgery.

Lewis and his parents discussed the merits of the new surgery. While most people with pectus excavatum never suffer any ill health effects, some research indicated the condition could possibly lead to lung or heart complications later in life. Although Lewis presently showed no signs of trouble, Helen and Bar worried that their son could have respiratory problems down the road if they did nothing. There was a surgeon who did the new procedure at a university teaching hospital located in South Carolina. They left the final decision about the surgery to Lewis and he opted to go through with the operation, reassured by his parents' belief that it was a safe procedure.

They finally made an appointment with the surgeon at the university hospital for September 15, 1999. However, the approach of hurricane Floyd led South Carolina's governor to evacuate coastal cities in South Carolina. Helen cancelled the trip at the last minute, and the family narrowly avoided spending 24 hours on a clogged highway, trying to escape potential disaster with thousands of other worried residents. Secretly, Helen wondered if it was some kind of omen.

When Lewis eventually saw the surgeon in October, the doctor agreed that Lewis was a good candidate for the procedure. It could be done in June the following year, after middle school let out and before high school began, a convenient time for a routine procedure. But as the time for the surgery drew closer there was another delay; the Blackman's health insurance provider refused to pay for the surgery, saying there was no proof it was necessary. Months of arguing followed between Helen and the insurance company, and her frustration grew. The surgeons at the hospital helped to convince the insurers that it was a matter of medical necessity, not merely cosmetic or experimental.

By the time the Blackman's insurance company relented and agreed to cover the costs, it was October of 2000. The surgeon wanted to perform the operation on a Monday, the day before Halloween, but Helen didn't think it was fair to make the children miss out on any holiday action. Halloween would be a last chance to have some fun before going into the hospital. They all settled on Thursday, November 2 as the date.

While Helen had the nurse on the phone to schedule the surgery, she asked her, "Shall I bring Lewis back down for another office visit with the doctor?" He must want to see Lewis, she thought. It's been an entire year since we were last there. Children change and grow, especially during their teens.

"It's not necessary…unless you just want to," replied the nurse. She explained that any tests or information could be handled when Lewis checked in the morning of the procedure. Helen was surprised, but took their word that it wouldn't add anything to what the surgeon needed to know. Besides, she didn't relish the idea of four hours in the car for such a brief visit.

Tuesday, October 31, 2000
With her mother's help, Eliza sewed her own Cleopatra costume for trick-or-treating. Far beyond such childish pastimes at his advanced age, Lewis was invited to a Halloween party with friends from his days in middle school. Although he loved being at Hammond and made plenty of new friends, he missed his childhood friends who had gone on to the public high school. Lewis had a great time that night, and felt it had been worth staying in town for an extra couple of days.

Wednesday, November 1
On Wednesday the family set out for the two-hour drive to the hospital. Along with the luggage, the car was fully loaded with snacks and juice boxes, and of course a large stash of Halloween candy from the night before. They looked like they were setting out on vacation as they pulled away from their comfortable gray brick bungalow.

Their room at the motel was dreary and cheerless, with stark regulation-issue furniture and a drab, impersonal decor. Helen hid her disappointment when they checked in and unpacked, although she wondered why the hospital's pediatric surgery department would recommend such an uninspiring place. They had told her the motel had an arrangement with the hospital, although a connection with the hospital was never mentioned by the hotel personnel. This room, this place, gave her an uneasy feeling she couldn't name.

Lewis had the honor of choosing where they ate dinner that night. He chose Poogan's Porch, a southern landmark known for their Lowcountry dishes, and located in a gracious, historic Victorian house. It was even rumored to be haunted by the home's original inhabitant. In a trip that was hardly a family holiday, this was the one part of the journey they had all looked forward to, and they celebrated being together.

Thursday, November 2

Accompanied by his family, Lewis checked in to the university's children's hospital at 6 a.m., with the surgery set to begin at 7:30. Besides his parents and sister, he brought an entire library of his favorite books for entertainment: the science fiction classic *Dune*, Shakespeare's play *Julius Caesar*, a book on the Israeli spy agency, the Mossaad, and several books from the bawdy *Flashman* series of historical comic novels about the British Empire. And, of course, he had his learner's permit.

A nurse asked Lewis how much he weighed instead of weighing him on a scale. Helen was disturbed by this, knowing that weight is how they determine the right dosage for drugs. She also knew that 15-year-old boys have egos, and suspected he might fudge the truth to appear larger and stronger. She insisted they weigh him, and found he had only 120 pounds on his 5-foot-4-inch frame, less than he admitted to.

As the nurses wheeled Lewis off to surgery, Helen told him she would be waiting when he awoke. She reminded him the surgery would be over in less than an hour.

The 45 minute time period they were told to expect for the procedure came and went, and Helen and Bar became increasingly concerned when two hours passed. This was supposed to be so simple, Helen thought. After another 30 minutes, the surgeon finally appeared in the waiting room to break the tension. He explained he had to reposition the metal bar in Lewis' chest four times to get it in the right position. But all in all, he told them, Lewis did fine.

Helen wondered if the doctor realized how much Lewis' chest depression had deepened since he last saw him a year ago. He hadn't laid eyes on Lewis again until the boy was in the operating room under anesthesia. Perhaps the doctor wasn't prepared for how severe it had become and it made the surgery more difficult.

In the recovery room Lewis was conscious and alert, and his vital signs were good. For pain control, he had an epidural line that infused narcotic painkillers into his back. When the nurses asked him to rate his pain on a 1-10 scale, he told them, "three." Good news. They also found he was fully oxygenated, the last time that would happen during his stay.

A large, burly man, tough-looking and built like a football linebacker, was in the next bed over, with the curtains partially drawn around him for privacy. He was beginning to come out of anesthesia, and was whining, "Owie, Owie," repeatedly in a high-pitched voice that sounded like a little girl with a skinned knee. As they listened to this, Lewis broke into an impish grin and looked over at his mother. The two of them exchanged knowing smiles at the touchingly childlike self-restraint of this powerful man. At least Helen knew that her son's sense of irony and compassion was intact.

The nurses and doctors in the recovery room noted that Lewis wasn't producing any urine and his Foley catheter was causing him pain. As Helen reconstructed it later, Lewis was apparently dehydrated from fasting for hours in preparation for the surgery, and although Lewis received IV fluids in the operating room, the chief surgical resident had written orders that reduced Lewis' fluids to a minimal amount after surgery. A nurse brought in a syringe of something to put in Lewis' IV line, and when Helen asked what it was, she was told Toradol. She had never heard of the drug and quizzed the nurse about what it was. The nurse explained it was medication they could use in conjunction with Lewis' narcotics to relieve post-operative pain, and it allowed them to use fewer opiates. That sounded like a positive thing to Helen. After a short time, Lewis began vomiting, and his skin was red and itchy. Despite this, he was taken upstairs to a room. He still had not urinated.

There were no rooms available in the surgical unit, so he was placed in the children's cancer ward for the time being. The family followed along to room 749. Lewis was still feeling ill and vomiting. He was receiving just enough liquid through his IV to keep his vein open. Bar took Eliza to get some food and go back to the motel for the night, while Helen stayed the night with Lewis in his room.

Friday, November 3

By Friday Lewis felt a little better, although he still suffered from some nausea and vomiting and had difficulty with pain control. The nurses continued to bring the syringes of Toradol every six hours. Helen stayed by Lewis' side and kept him company, supervising his care and helping to take his mind off his discomfort. Late Friday, after his IV fluids were adjusted to an appropriate amount, he finally began urinating, to Helen's enormous relief.

She learned from overhearing the staff that they were preparing for an upcoming inspection by the Joint Commission, a hospital accrediting organization. Everything had to be in order for next week's visit. At the time, Helen looked on it only as an interesting piece of workplace gossip or trivia that she picked up by being a temporary visitor in their world.

Lewis' surgeon left on Friday night to begin his weekend. Helen began another night of fitful napping in room 749 with her son.

Saturday, November 4

On Saturday morning at 9:00, another doctor from Lewis' surgeon's office stopped in to check on Lewis during rounds. He found Lewis to be making satisfactory progress and wrote in his patient chart. *No evidence of infection. Clear lungs. May sit up and consider getting out of bed.* When this doctor left after examining Lewis, Helen had no idea that he would be the last experienced physician she and her son would see for the next two days.

By evening, Lewis developed a slight fever and his feet felt cold to the touch. Helen thought he should be improving and feeling better by now.

Sunday, November 5

Lewis and Helen awoke at 6 a.m. sharp when a nurse came to deliver yet another dose of Toradol. Just 30 minutes later Lewis gasped and held his breath. Through clenched teeth, he tried to tell his mother he had terrible pain in his upper abdomen. She asked him how bad it was.

"It's the worst pain imaginable," he whispered, barely able to speak. Helen summoned a nurse with the call button.

The nurse asked Lewis to describe his pain on a scale. "Five on a scale of five," he replied in amazement, as if he couldn't quite believe it himself. It was clear to Helen that he was in agony. Three days after surgery he should be improving, not suffering mysterious new pains. And why did it hurt in his upper abdomen when the surgery was performed on his chest?

The night shift nurse seemed alarmed and left the room. A few minutes later she bustled back in and announced that it was just "gas pains", and that nothing could be done. In most circumstances, the sudden onset of such intense pain would cause nurses to alert an attending physician, an experienced veteran doctor, to examine the patient. Helen thought it odd that the night nurse had a change in her concern so suddenly, as if another person had convinced her not to be alarmed. It was the change of shift and Helen later pondered as to if the day nurse coming on duty had ill advised the night nurse not to worry and that Lewis' pain was only "gas pains". "There's nothing I can do for gas pains." She wrote in his chart - *Gas pains, patient needs to move around.*

The day nurse who came on duty appeared to be indifferent and insensitive to Lewis' deteriorating condition. This Sunday was to be the pivotal point for Lewis who needed desperately to be rescued and not ignored or placated. Unbeknown to Helen, the life raft for rescue would be obscured from Lewis' reach by the actions of one nurse.

Later, the day nurse came in and suggested a bath might help Lewis to feel more comfortable. The nurse urged Lewis to sit up in a chair after bathing, but he appeared even weaker than before. It was like climbing Mt. Everest to get him into that chair. After Helen finally maneuvered him painfully into the seat, Lewis was exhausted. He said, "I think this was a mistake," meaning he was too weak and nauseated to either sit up or get back in the bed. Helen said fervently, "I think so, too," meaning it was a mistake ever to have the surgery. Then Helen realized that even at this terrible moment that her sensible son was only looking forward, trying to solve the problem at hand, how to get back in the bed.

When all this failed to help, the day nurse insisted that Lewis' pain could only be improved by "ambulating." When Lewis was too weak to stand unassisted, the nurse and Helen half-dragged him around the ward, with Lewis stopping to rest on Helen's shoulder every two or three steps. The nurse admonished Lewis for being sluggish and lazy. The nurse wrote in Lewis' chart - *Does not understand the importance of ambulation.*

In a continued attempt to ease his pain, the nurses kept up the regular injections of Toradol. But by Sunday afternoon Lewis' abdomen hurt worse than ever, and he was still unable to keep even small amounts of water down. His belly grew rigid and distended, and his eyes had a sunken, hollow look. Helen noticed his skin was pale and felt clammy. Droplets of cold sweat covered his face and made his hair damp, and his temperature had dropped.

Alarmed by his condition, Helen thought that Lewis needed to see a doctor as soon as possible. She repeatedly pushed the call button, but they had stopped answering the call light in room 749. Helen suspected they had decided she was a nuisance. Some of them had gone to the break room. Outside in the hallway she could hear other nurses and aides decorating the ward and chatting. They were primping and polishing for the big hospital inspection next day.

Lewis gripped Helen's hand like it was a lifeline and he was drowning. She could tell how intense his pain was from the way he clutched at her with what little remaining strength he had. The sound of laughter floated down the hall from the staff break room, and seemed grotesquely out of place when her son was suffering such torture. How helpless it felt to see your child like this and be unable to do something for him.

Using the call light and intercom, Helen repeatedly asked that a doctor be sent to take a look at Lewis. After several requests, she realized that there was some connection between her asking for a doctor, and the appearance, some time later, of a rumpled, exhausted-looking young intern who did not see anything wrong with Lewis. Helen was concerned. She had assumed they would send someone experienced. What she got was a young intern with a brand-new degree from a college of osteopathic medicine, although no one revealed that at the time. But clearly this woman they sent was not what Helen had in mind.

Helen walked out to the nurses' station, weary and frustrated, to find no nurse there. She followed the sound of cheerful voices to the nurses' break room and again asked the nurse to call in another physician. The day nurse argued with Helen, telling her she had just seen a doctor, as if that should be good enough to satisfy her. Helen asked by name for another physician on call. The nurse wrote in Lewis' chart - *Parent requesting upper level M.D.* The time was 6:26 in the evening.

This time the intern came quickly. Both the nurse and the intern seemed insulted and exasperated by Helen's insistence on having someone with more experience. In desperation, Helen reviewed the frightening set of symptoms her son was exhibiting.

"Can't you see his pallor and the dark circles under his eyes? He's in a cold sweat, he has severe abdominal pain that never stops," Helen recounted. The intern nodded silently, never uttering a word. Helen thought the doctor was too angry to speak.

At last the chief resident came to Lewis's room at 8 p.m., and Helen assumed he was the veteran doctor she'd been asking for. He didn't wear a name tag that indicated what his exact title was, so it wasn't clear that he was a fourth-year resident and not an attending physician. Helen was at the mercy of her own naïve trust. Tall and handsome, this young doctor was fashionably dressed and had an air of confidence. He was wearing a jacket and brought a whiff of cold night air with him. It was a startling reminder that time was passing in the world outside. When Lewis had entered the hospital, it was Indian summer. He had been wearing shorts and sandals. Helen felt as though they had been in that little room forever.

When he checked Lewis, the chief resident made a diagnosis of a blocked intestine and he ordered a suppository to ease the blockage. He wrote on the chart - *Probable ileus*. He also noted on the chart that Lewis' heart rate was in the 80s, although a nurse during that same time recorded his heart rate at 126 beats-per-minute. Helen asked the doctor about the sweating and lowered temperature, now at 97.7 degrees, but he dismissed the symptoms as side effects of the other medication that Lewis was taking. A metabolic panel was ordered on Lewis' blood that night, but no one thought to order a simple complete blood count (CBC) to check for bleeding or infection. Now that Helen believed Lewis had been seen by a veteran doctor, she no longer pestered the staff to send someone else. She was still worried about Lewis, but she thought since he had seen an attending physician, she had gone as high up the ladder as possible.

Suppositories and medications failed to help Lewis that night. His pain never eased and his condition deteriorated as the hours wore on. Helen kept her sleepless vigil Sunday night, trying to help Lewis hang on until the regular weekday staff and doctors returned. She felt like they were lost in the wilderness waiting to be rescued.

Helen waited for the tide to turn. At midnight, his heart rate was 142, and his temperature was only 95 degrees. By 4 a.m. his temperature stood at 96.6 and his heart was beating 140 times-per-minute. Helen had never seen an intensive care unit, but instinctively felt that Lewis' current doctors and nurses were not capable of caring for a patient in his condition. She thought he must belong in the ICU, but she hadn't a clue about how to get him there.

Monday, November 6
As morning broke, the awful pain in Lewis' abdomen abruptly stopped. When the resident heard this news, she took it as a positive sign and said, "Oh, good." But to Helen it seemed strange, like the eerie calm in the eye of a hurricane, where things are temporarily quiet before even greater trouble lands onshore.

A parade of residents marched through Lewis' room in those first hours of the day. Helen asked the second year residents what she thought about Lewis' pale color; his lips looked as if they had lost all pigment and were the same color as his face. The cheerful resident was unconcerned and told her it was just the result of low blood pressure—nothing to worry about.

When an aide came at 8:30 and attempted to take Lewis' vital signs, she was unable to find any blood pressure. Instead of calling for an attending physician, for the next two hours aides and nurses tried and failed to take his blood pressure with various cuffs, assuming that the equipment was faulty. They wrapped cuffs around both arms and both legs, trying different devices each time, but with no results. By 10:30 they had given up, but still no one called for a veteran doctor. A day nurse wrote on Lewis' chart - *Unable to obtain B.P.….B.P. attempts on arms and legs unsuccessful.* By then Lewis' father, Bar, had come with Eliza in tow.

Before noon, an x-ray technician arrived in Lewis' room with a portable machine to get some films of his abdomen. Lewis was by now so weak he could not get out of bed. In spite of his weakened state, Lewis tried to cooperate with the technician, working with him to find a position he could tolerate so the technician could still take the pictures he needed. Lewis was directing the process, and the effort to get into position for the x-rays strained his body to the breaking point.

As the x-ray technician packed up his equipment, someone from the lab came to take a blood sample. No amount of squeezing or pressure helped any longer to extract blood from Lewis, and at that point he began to black out. Helen was standing next to the bed and Lewis tried to speak, but his speech was labored and slurred.

"Ish going black." He then repeated it once more, "Ish going black." When he said this, the x-ray and lab technicians took advantage of the moment to scurry away, racing down the hall and away from the scene as quickly as possible. No one offered to get a doctor or give any aid. Lewis was in cardiac arrest.

Helen ran out into the hallway, frantic, yelling, "He's seizing, he's seizing!" She found the chief resident near the nurses' station and together they rushed back into the room.

The chief resident stood by the bed for two minutes, shouting Lewis' name to see if he would respond. The family looked on as he called loudly, "Lewis! Lewis!"

"We'll have to ask you all to leave," the chief resident said calmly. "We're going to have to do a procedure." He motioned for Helen and Bar to take Eliza and go out to the hallway. Procedure…what procedure? Helen later learned from the medical record that the resident had put chest tubes in Lewis, before resuscitating him. An earlier X-ray had shown a small amount of air pressing on Lewis' lung and the young doctor had surmised that this was causing his symptoms. In fact, it was a typical side effect of the chest surgery Lewis had undergone. It was not the cause of Lewis' cardiac arrest.

A code was called, fifteen minutes after Lewis went into cardiac arrest, and at last the staff rushed to Lewis' room. Surgeons and equipment converged on room 749 as if it was the center of the universe. Helen couldn't help thinking, where were they yesterday? For an hour they worked, sparing no effort or tools. Nurses hooked up new IV lines, doctors performed cardiopulmonary resuscitation, and they shocked him with a defibrillator repeatedly.

Helen, Bar and Eliza stood in the hallway, dumbstruck and numb. When Helen turned around, a hospital chaplain was standing behind her and she recoiled in horror. "Don't worry, I come to all the codes." She believed him. It was impossible to think that anything terrible could really happen to her vibrant, healthy boy. The entire scenario felt surreal.

But it had already happened. Lewis could not be revived. Doctors recorded the time of death at 1:23 p.m. on Monday, November 6, nearly 31 hours after Lewis began having stomach pains.

Someone came out to get them. Helen feared that they were going to tell her Lewis was now disabled or brain-damaged. They were taken into a room with a total of five surgeons, each wearing green hospital scrubs. A man introduced himself to Helen and Bar as Dr. Lopez, the doctor on call. Why had they never seen him before? Dr. Lopez simply said, "We lost him."

"What do you mean, 'lost him?'" Helen asked. She didn't understand what he meant. It made no sense to her. Dr. Lopez had to repeat it several more times before it began to register. Lewis wasn't battling an illness; he came in a healthy boy. How could they "lose" him? Helen and Bar sat in stunned silence without crying. To cry, they would have had to believe this unimaginable event actually happened. It made no sense to them.

The only words that would come out of Helen's mouth were,

"What happened?"

Dr. Lopez had little to offer Helen and Bar. "Lewis' death is a mystery. Our chief resident found nothing wrong the night before."

For the first time, Helen realized the self-confident young man who had been treating Lewis the night before was not the experienced doctor she requested so many times; he was only a resident. Later, Helen's shock and grief would be mixed with anger and a feeling of betrayal. But for now, she was too numb. Dr. Lopez asked permission to do an autopsy, and Helen followed her knee-jerk reaction and told him no. She didn't want the hospital hurting her son any more.

Bar and Helen began the horrible task of calling relatives and friends to tell them about Lewis. All the advice they heard, some of it from relatives in the medical field, said to get an autopsy. They called the hospital and requested one as soon as possible.

Helen hadn't stayed at the motel since that first night before the surgery; she spent all her time in the hospital with Lewis. Now she was staying there waiting for the autopsy to be performed in the morning. She knew sleep wouldn't come that night. To be back in the dreary little motel room, knowing that her innocent child was lying in the morgue a few blocks away, was like being in Hell. They had packed up Lewis' things that afternoon, everything he brought except his brand new learner's permit. It was missing and they couldn't find it anywhere.

The autopsy report showed Lewis bled to death internally from a perforated ulcer, caused by the repeated doses of Toradol. A child of Lewis' size has a total of four to five liters of blood, and his abdomen was filled with roughly three liters of blood and digestive fluid. Lewis had lost up to 75 percent of his entire blood supply into his abdominal cavity.

10%

PERCENTAGE OF NON-NARCOTIC ANALGESIC RELATED MEDICATION ERRORS THAT RESULT IN SERIOUS PATIENT HARM

21%

PERCENTAGE OF NARCOTIC ANALGESIC RELATED MEDICATION ERRORS THAT RESULT IN SERIOUS PATIENT HARM

Lewis' surgeon called Helen and Bar to tell them about the perforated ulcer. A month later, they returned to the surgeon's office to meet with him. When Helen told him how hard she tried to get the staff to listen, to send for an experienced doctor for Lewis, the surgeon apologized and told them Lewis' death could have been prevented. Helen figured the nurses and residents were all in over their heads, but just didn't want to bother anybody, and that's why they failed. They were more afraid of upsetting a superior than of hurting a patient.

"We have something in the South called the 'Yo Mama rule,'" Helen says in a honeyed drawl. "Would you give 'Yo Mama' that treatment? They forgot that rule."

AND ALL THE DAYS TO COME

Returning home to Columbia was indescribable for the family. The entire series of events was incomprehensible, so bizarre and totally unexpected. One by one, each member of the family peeked into Lewis' bedroom, thinking somehow maybe he would be there. "I didn't know *where* he was," Helen later said.

Bar and Helen made a pallet on their bedroom floor for Eliza to sleep on, so she wouldn't be alone at night. Helen wasn't able to bear reading anything but children's books. She would burrow under the covers of her bed and read Harry Potter or Lemony Snicket to Eliza. It was at least a week before she could bring herself to clean out the family car. When she finally did, there were the candy wrappers and CDs and snacks, "Just like a vacation," she said. "Just like always, except Lewis never came home."

Helen expected to be contacted by the hospital after Lewis died. She and her husband thought there would be an investigation, but they never contacted her.

The community rallied behind them, and friends and neighbors provided support and help. Eliza went back to her small Montessori school, but her misery was compounded when her friends and classmates fell into an awkward silence whenever she mentioned her brother. Helen never went back to finish her Ph.D., and instead became an advocate for patients' rights, founding Mothers Against Medical Errors (MAME), a grassroots organization working to change laws that involve patient safety. Bar retired a short time later, and he makes it possible for Helen to do her work on behalf of others.

Eventually a settlement was reached with the hospital over Lewis' case. Part of the money went to fund college scholarships in Lewis' name, at Hammond and at Dreher High School in Columbia. Part of the money went toward the Lewis Blackman youth company at the South Carolina Shakespeare Company. Another portion went to build a campers' center called Blackman Commons at Camp Greenville, Lewis' summer camp in the North Carolina Mountains. Much of the rest went to patient safety efforts in Lewis' name.

But even when you go on, Helen knows, life is never the same. "All the metaphors you hear about losing a child are true. When Lewis died, it was like a part of me had been torn out. It was like a giant cleaver in our lives."

Her greatest sadness is the loss of Lewis' future promise. "My biggest regrets are all the things he never got to do. He never fell in love. He never traveled, the thing he wanted most in the world," according to Helen. "When he was little and we read an atlas, I would tell him as much as I knew about all the places in the world that he could someday visit. I had filled him with a yearning to see the world, but in the end he never even rode on an airplane."

Lewis received a total of 17 adult-dose injections of Toradol between Thursday, November 2 and Monday, November 6. Toradol is a potent non-steroidal anti-inflammatory drug (NSAID) that carries special risks and requires careful monitoring.

31%

PERCENTAGE OF MEDICATION ERRORS THAT RESULT FROM ADMINISTRATION OF THE WRONG DOSE FOR A PRESCRIBED DRUG

- Toradol is banned in five European countries, and is used with very tight restrictions in most other countries where it is permitted.
- Toradol is not recommended in repeated doses for children and adolescents under 16.
  - This limit was set by a label change in 2002, two years after Lewis' death.
- Repeated dosages of Toradol can cause an elevated risk of serious gastro-intestinal bleeding and kidney damage.
- A minority of patients suffer allergic reactions to Toradol.
- The pharmaceutical company that manufactures Toradol, stipulates that patients receiving the drug should be carefully monitored for adverse reactions.

1 in 17

MEDICATION ERRORS THAT ARE AS A RESULT OF WRONG DOSES RESULTING IN PATIENT HARM REQUIRING TREATMENT

The potent dosage administered to Lewis caused a hole to form in his intestines which began to bleed. Blood and digestive fluids seeped directly into his abdominal cavity over the weekend. By Monday afternoon, Lewis had lost significant body fluid, and this led to a complete collapse of his circulatory system.

Beginning as early as Saturday evening, Lewis began showing signs of early deterioration. Post-operative shock is most often caused by blood loss or infection. Lewis exhibited telltale symptoms of shock that should have alerted healthcare providers early, only if they had listened and examined the patient in their care. Lewis had these symptoms:

- Pallor and lack of color in his lips
- Rapid pulse rate
- Cold, clammy skin and profuse sweating
- Shallow, labored breathing
- Lethargy and faintness
- Unexplained abdominal pain

All of these were initial clues, and the sudden onset of abdominal pain was a classic sign that Lewis was in trouble. Patients can occasionally have pain in an area different from the surgical site, known as referred pain, or they may have gas pockets from anesthesia. But any prolonged, intense pain must be thoroughly evaluated and tested to find the cause.

Lewis' attending physician and surgeon, signed off care to a resident physician on Sunday. A resident is a licensed physician, but is still in a stage of postgraduate medical training. Although residency programs provide intensive training, residents are inexperienced physicians. Helen thought the resident who saw Lewis on Sunday night was a veteran doctor. She didn't recognize and was not clearly told that this was a fourth-year resident. After repeatedly asking for help, she thought an experienced physician had been called and Lewis would receive much-needed care.

These varying levels of physicians can be confusing to patients and their families. More often than not, doctors, nurses and technicians don't introduce themselves or explain their role. During any hospital stay, there can be a host of healthcare professionals in and out of a patient's room. In a teaching hospital, there are significantly more levels of physicians, residents and medical students caring for a patient. The doctor who is responsible for a patient's care is known as the attending physician. An attending is a physician who has completed residency, and practices medicine in a hospital, usually focusing on a specialty learned during residency and/or a fellowship program. An attending physician may supervise residents, interns and medical students. Legally, attending physicians have the final responsibility for patient care.

Lewis needed intervention and did not receive it. His case illustrates several key fatal points:

- Staff and physicians failed to listen and hear what Lewis was saying, and his mother's pleas were ignored.
- Staff and physicians failed to recognize the classic signs of shock.
- Staff failed to contact Lewis' surgeon during the weekend.
- Physicians failed to order the most useful and basic blood test, a blood count (CBC) or perform an "abdominal, peritoneal tap" at his bedside to quickly and conclusively determine intra-abdominal bleeding.

The family instinctively recognized a change in Lewis' condition, but they were not clinical experts and were not equipped to identify the root cause of his symptoms. The nurses and residents should have heeded the warnings and his progressively deteriorating state. They needed to take action or contact a higher level physician, such as the attending physician or another surgeon, regardless of what day or time it was.

While many medical errors are caused by a cascade of system failures, this error was a fundamental failure of not hearing or listening to a patient. This failure to listen or respond to the patient and family is a key weakness in our system. There is evidence, from both research and observation, that poor communication with patients has become prevalent in healthcare. Patients who ask too many questions are looked at as annoying or even difficult. When Helen went to the nurses' station for help, her requests were viewed as bothersome.

There are other similar documented cases where patients have tried to warn doctors and nurses that they were making a mistake, but no one listened to the patient. One study in a large academic medical center, not unlike the one where Lewis was a patient, found that communication failures contributed to error. In an article written in the Annals of Internal Medicine (Chassim & Becher), the authors reviewed a case where a patient received a cardiac catheterization procedure intended for another patient, despite telling the doctors and nurses they were making a mistake. The principles of not listening were the cause of performing the procedure on the wrong patient. The authors noted:

> "Perhaps the most striking feature of this case—one that will be familiar to all clinicians who have worked in large hospitals—is the frighteningly poor communication it exemplifies. Physicians failed to communicate with nurses, attending physicians failed to communicate with residents and fellows, staff from one unit failed to communicate with those from others, and no one listened carefully to the patient. Although no data exists to document how widespread communication failures are, they are probably endemic in large, complex academic medical centers."

Some of these same principles apply in Lewis' case. Healthcare professionals are taught to assess and listen to their patients. Nonetheless, the actual practice is not consistently followed. These professionals have a broad base of knowledge and experience that has no doubt helps many patients. Even so, a fatal assumption occurs when healthcare professionals take the posture that, "we know what's best." This can be a recipe for disaster when it results in ignoring important information. The patient usually knows a great deal about their illness, medicines and treatments. Often the patient is the first one to know that something is "different", and when the patient says that something is wrong, they should be heard.

So why did the clinicians all miss the signs that Lewis was in trouble? Lewis' surgeon later said,

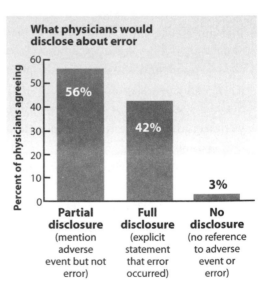

What physicians would disclose about error

Percent of physicians agreeing

- Partial disclosure (mention adverse event but not error): 56%
- Full disclosure (explicit statement that error occurred): 42%
- No disclosure (no reference to adverse event or error): 3%

Source: Gallagher TH, Garbutt FM, Waterman AD, et al. Choosing your words carefully: how physicians would disclose harmful medical errors to patients. Arch Intern Med. 2006; 166:1585-1593

"He broke the rule." What he meant was that Lewis did not exhibit the classic symptoms like vomiting blood or passing blood from his intestine, and because he was bleeding into his abdominal cavity, the seriousness of his condition was missed.

But other experts say the warning signs were evident, stating Lewis' symptoms should have been recognized and treated. A group of medical experts, who later reviewed Lewis' medical records for attorney Richard Gergel, helped him summarize the case.

"This is about a boy who bled to death over 30 hours, in a hospital with modern technology and vast technical resources," said the attorney reviewer. "Our experts' main point was that Lewis wasn't properly monitored."

The reviewing attorney went on to point out that, given Lewis' symptoms, an experienced doctor would have known to order a routine blood test, a complete blood count (CBC), that would have shown Lewis was bleeding internally. "The test costs about $30," he said. "Our experts couldn't understand why it wasn't ordered. It's one of the most common tests in hospitals."

After Lewis' death, Helen also sent his records to another physician, a friend and former assistant professor who taught at several university hospitals medical schools. He is a veteran anesthesiologist who has taught hundreds of medical students, and participated in thousands of surgical procedures. The doctor was appalled by what he saw.

"Even a Boy Scout could have done better," he claimed. "It's hard to kill a healthy 15-year-old." The doctor believes Lewis probably could have been saved up through Monday morning.

MOVING FORWARD

Helen Haskell has chosen to use the tragic loss of her son to benefit others, and has had a big impact on patient safety. Helen has worked with South Carolina legislators to enact the Lewis Blackman Hospital Patient Safety Act. The state law mandates South Carolina hospitals to comply with certain provisions:

- Upon admission, hospitals must inform patients in writing of their right to contact their attending physician directly, and provide a mechanism for the patient or family to make contact promptly.

- Advise patients of the right to request a higher level clinical staff member to intervene in patient care and provide a means for patients to call for assistance in the hospital.
- All hospital staff must wear name badges clearly stating their position and ranking.

All of these factors might have helped Lewis' family to take additional action, if they had access to this same information when he was a patient

In addition to enacting the Lewis Blackman Hospital Patient Safety Act, Helen founded Mothers Against Medical Errors (MAME). The group is active in improving patient safety and providing support to other families and their experiences with medical errors.

PROTECT YOURSELF IN TODAY'S HEALTHCARE SYSTEM

Rapid Response Teams: A new approach used to respond to patients like Lewis, called Rapid Response Team (RRT), or Medical Emergency Team (MET), has been developed and implemented at many hospitals over the last five years. Even though there is controversial or questionable evidence in the peer-reviewed medical literature regarding the impact of RRTs on averting preventable medical error deaths, conceptually it is the right thing to have in place to further safeguard the environment of care for patients.

An effective Rapid Response Team (RRT) brings critical care expertise to the bedside of the decompensating patient promptly so that a life can be saved.

- A patient showing signs of worsening blood pressure, pulse rate, fever, pain or breathing problems are evaluated by an RRT made up of critical care nurses, technicians and doctors.
- Any staff member can call the rescue team, including an aide or technician. No staff member is to be reprimanded for calling the

team, even if the patient was not in distress.

- Hospital's can also provide an avenue for a family member to request an RRT intervention, if they feel adequate help has not been received.

- The concept is to treat the patient long before they become critical or have a code situation like the one Lewis experienced.

These rescue teams are growing across the nation. The University Health System Consortium (UHC) is an alliance of 97 academic medical centers and 149 of their affiliated hospitals, representing nearly 90 percent of the nation's non-profit academic medical centers. The UHC fully supports and recommends the use of Rapid Response Teams (RRT) in their member hospitals. UHC has found that failure to recognize the clinically unstable patient outside of the ICU setting is a major cause of greater than expected mortality.

Seven years after Lewis' death, the hospital where he died started a Medical Emergency Team (MET). Helen Haskell said, "Rapid Response Teams are the most significant innovation in the patient safety movement. People assume that when they are in a hospital, they'll be monitored. But outside of the emergency room and intensive care unit, most hospitals aren't set up to deal with emergencies." Unfortunately, many hospitals have not put these teams in place.

- If you are checking into a hospital for treatment or surgery, ask what the process is for reporting an error or a concern.

- Find out if your hospital has a Rapid Response Team or Medical Emergency Team in place.

REPORTING SAFETY CONCERNS WHILE IN THE HOSPITAL

Beginning in 2007, the Joint Commission, an organization that evaluates and accredits most hospitals in the United States, now requires a mechanism for hospitalized patients to report concerns regarding safety.

- Hospitals must encourage patients' active involvement in their own care as a patient safety strategy.

- Hospitals must define and communicate the means for patients and their families to report concerns about safety, and encourage them to do so.
- Check to see if your local hospital has a mechanism in place for this and ask them to describe the process.

MEDICATIONS AND WEIGHT

It is critical to be aware of any medications a child or teenager is receiving in the hospital. Lewis' weight needed to be carefully considered before administering Toradol. The attending physician, surgeon, residents, pharmacists and nurses may have had opportunities to review the dose calculation when caring for Lewis. The number of injections Lewis received exceeded the drug label's recommendations. But no healthcare professional questioned this high dose or prolonged use.

2-3 million

NUMBER OF HOSPITALIZED PATIENTS EVERY YEAR THAT HAVE A MEDICATION ERROR

3

THE NUMBER OF TIMES THAT ADVERSE DRUG EVENTS ARE MORE FREQUENT IN CHILDREN COMPARED TO ADULTS

- Find out if the physician and pharmacist have carefully considered the child's weight, and if the medication dose matches the child's weight.
- Ask if the weight adjusted dose has been confirmed by the nurses administering the medication.

STATE PATIENT SAFETY ACTS

Individual states can have vastly different laws regarding patient safety. It benefits patients and their families to be well informed about the laws in the state where they receive treatment.

- Find out if your state has a patient safety act. What does it say, and is it enforced at your local hospitals?
- Write to your legislators and ask what they have done for patient safety in your state or local community.
- Find out if your regional area has a patient safety consortium which consists of local hospitals working together to improve safety. Ask if they have a community chapter for consumer input.
- Most of all, if you are in an uncomfortable situation in a hospital, clinic or other healthcare setting, do not be afraid to speak up and get help until your issue is resolved. It is your right.

TODAY

According to Helen on the role of the support group she founded, Mothers Against Medical Errors, "I view MAME's role as providing support to medical error victims and advocating for causes that improve patient safety. In South Carolina, legislation has been a big part of that. We have been closely involved in two other pieces of legislation after the Lewis Blackman Act: a hospital infection disclosure act, which passed in 2006, and a heart patient safety act, which we are working on now." No doubt these efforts will help to prevent other medical errors.

Until medical errors can be significantly reduced through progressive systems improvements, culture of safety infusion, what you do and say may save your life or a loved one the next time you are in a hospital.

When you are admitted to a hospital ask about:
- Which physician will be in charge of your care?
- How can you contact the physician directly if needed?
- Who will be covering for them if they are unavailable and how can they be reached?
- Does the hospital have a Rapid Response Team (RRT) or MET in place?

Promote good communication by:
- Asking each healthcare worker involved with your care to introduce themselves.
- Ask for each healthcare worker's position and title and, if necessary, ask for clarification.
- Be alert of worker's name tags.
- *Immediately inform healthcare workers about any symptoms that appear following a procedure or after receiving medication of any kind*

You have the right to:
- Question any medication, treatment or procedure.
- Ask for additional information about why a medication, treatment or procedure is needed.
- Refuse a medication, treatment or procedure.
- Ask for assistance from a higher level of help to resolve a situation.
- To use the chain of command and get additional help regarding your care.
- To refuse care from interns and residents and only receive care from an attending physician or surgeon.

Going up the "care" chain:
- If your concern is not addressed, ask to speak to the chief of the related department, such as pediatrics, obstetrics and gynecology, cardiology, etc.
- If the issue is still not resolved, insist on speaking to the Chief of Staff or Chief Medical Officer.

CHAPTER 2

READING BETWEEN

In this chapter
- Find out the importance of a second opinion and how to get one.
- Discover when it's smart to have a lab specimen analyzed by a second laboratory.
- Learn how to use the Internet to empower yourself with information, and how it can change the course of your treatment.
- When you're uncomfortable with a diagnosis or a recommended treatment, what should you do?

*Why are "**misdiagnosis errors**" important for you to know about?*
Misdiagnosis can be devastating, leading to unnecessary treatment and medication for a condition or disease the patient doesn't have. It is estimated that each year thousands of Americans are mistakenly told they have the wrong condition. If not corrected quickly, a misdiagnosis can start a domino effect, subjecting healthy people to procedures, medications or treatments they don't need, while the real problem progresses or goes unchecked.

THE LINES

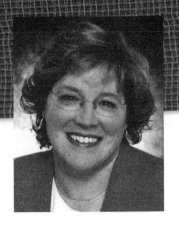

Trisha Torrey

Trisha Torrey hung up the phone, her eyes glazed over with disbelief as she stared across her bedroom. "Lymphoma," she repeated the word to herself in a quiet whisper. All the common associations galloped through her head - cancer, malignancy, terminal. This couldn't be right. She looked down at the piece of paper she held in her hand, where she had written the words as her surgeon, Dr. Andrews, said them - "Subcutaneous Paniculitis-like T-Cell Lymphoma." What a long, strange name.

When the surgeon removed the lump in Trisha's side at his office, it had never occurred to her that it might be cancer. The lump just appeared one day. She remembered watering the impatiens and daisies along her front walkway on that hot day in June. Her arm brushed against her torso as she wrestled with the garden hose, and she felt something that interrupted the normal contours of her body. There it was on her upper abdomen, under the skin and shaped like a golf ball. It wasn't even painful.

After palpating the lump with her fingers, she set down the hose and made a beeline for the phone to call her doctor's office. Trisha wasn't an alarmist, but she was a woman who believed in taking care of things that needed her attention. Calling Dr. Charles' office, she explained to his nurse what she had found and what it looked like. The nurse worked Trisha into his busy schedule for the next day.

From there it all happened so quickly. There was little time to think or ask questions. Dr. Charles examined the lump during Trisha's appointment, and immediately arranged for her to visit a surgeon, Dr. Andrews, the same day. She was surprised by his urgency to take care of it so soon. That afternoon in the surgeon's office Trisha felt a mixture of nervousness and relief; she didn't relish the thought of a biopsy, but she was glad to be getting this over with so she could have some peace of mind.

Dr. Andrews numbed the area, and before she knew it the procedure was finished. Just like that, Trisha thought - it was easier than getting my teeth cleaned. She hadn't wanted to watch the procedure or see the lump after it was removed, but now that it was done her curiosity overpowered her squeamishness.

"May I see it?" she asked the doctor, hoping she wouldn't be sorry once she got a look at it.

"It's already gone," Dr. Andrews told her as his nurse finished packing the specimen. The nurse slipped out quickly, carrying the offending lump with her.

Trisha wanted to know what the surgeon thought it was, and to her surprise he told her he had never seen anything like it before. She didn't find his words reassuring.

"I got it all, the entire lump," he said confidently. "I'll be sending the specimen over to the lab, and I'll call you as soon as we have the results. Of course," he cautioned her, "the results might be delayed because of the upcoming Fourth-of-July weekend. But when I know something I'll get in touch with you.

Trisha wondered how she would wait for answers through the holiday weekend and beyond. That evening she combed the web for any information she could find, beginning with search terms like "lump" and "tumor." As a successful self-employed marketing professional she often designed websites for clients, and understood better than most how to do an effective Internet search. She learned a lot, but in the absence of a diagnosis it was a futile exercise.

One week later, Trisha returned to Dr. Andrews' office to have her stitches removed. She felt optimistic and figured, since they hadn't called, that while she was there they would probably tell her that everything checked out fine. The doctor commented how well her incision was healing, but Trisha was anxious and needed emotional reassurance. She asked about the pathology report and was told it wasn't back yet. Another week passed and there was no call from Dr. Andrews, so she phoned his office only to find they still had no results.

Despite her anxiety, life flowed on while she was waiting. The home remodel she had started, a major undertaking, was moving along. Deciding the cozy raised ranch would be her permanent home for years to come, Trisha had begun the project to make it her dream house. Her girls were grown and she lived alone with her dog, so she could tailor it to please herself as she liked. There would be a gourmet kitchen, a hot tub and a luxurious bathroom where she could relax. A wall was now torn out between the kitchen and another room, giving a whole new meaning to the term "great-room." Electrical wires hung out in plain sight, and dust from sheetrock settled on counter tops and furniture. But it wasn't enough to keep her from having her weekly family dinners.

On Thursday, July 15, Trisha planned a family dinner with her parents and her daughters, as she did every week. Her mother suffered from Alzheimer's disease, and the weekly family dinners at Trisha's house gave her father a good home-cooked meal and a much-needed social outing with her mom. Becca and Ashley, Trisha's twenty-something daughters, shared an apartment nearby, and the family evenings also were an excuse to catch up with her girls' busy lives.

The phone rang around seven that evening, just as they all sat down to eat. As she headed for the bedroom to answer the phone, she told everyone to go ahead and start without her. When she picked up, Dr. Andrews' voice was on the other end of the line.

"Sorry it took so long for the results," he said in a deadpan, business-like tone. "Two independent lab tests confirmed *Subcutaneous Panniculitis-like T-cell Lymphoma* . . ." Trisha stopped hearing much of what the doctor said after that.

The brief call ended and she braced herself to go back out to the kitchen. Rejoining the group at the dinner table, Trisha managed to paste a neutral look on her face. She looked around at her family and her gaze fell on her mother. For the first time, she was glad her mother was lost in the maze of Alzheimer's. She wouldn't have to feel the pain of her daughter's diagnosis. Most days she didn't even know she had a daughter. Trisha could only think about getting them all out of the house so she could begin investigating her disease. Usually the evening flew by, but tonight the minutes dragged on as the pressure to know more grew inside of her.

At 9:30 that night, she hugged her family good-bye and

immediately went online. This time she had something to work with. Subcutaneous Panniculitis-like T-cell Lymphoma, or SPTCL for short. Her fingers flew over the keyboard searching every potential lead on the Internet she could find. There were hundreds of webpage links on lymphoma, but unfortunately she found precious little that was specifically about SPTCL. The limited information she did find was not encouraging.

The first Web link stated, "SPTCL is an uncommon type of cutaneous lymphoma with an aggressive natural history. It generally carries a poor prognosis despite standard anthracycline-based chemotherapy." The next link revealed the same prognosis, as did almost every other link she visited. Trisha stayed up all night hoping the next article she read would have a different outcome, a brighter forecast. By morning she was a wreck, her eyes bloodshot and her wavy brown hair disheveled. Although her mind continued churning and she was still confused, now she was determined to battle whatever this was.

Now that she had a better idea of what she was up against, her first order of business was telling her family over the weekend. Her father took the news with grace. "It's not a death sentence," he reminded her. "I survived prostate cancer. You'll get through this."

Becca and Ashley offered support, showing surprising maturity and strength. Here was their chance to help their mother, repaying her for everything she'd done for them while they were growing up. Trisha swore her family to secrecy because she didn't want clients to shy away from her business when they heard the word "cancer." She needed the income, especially now that the future looked so uncertain. She put the home remodel on hold for the time being. Who knew if the money would be needed elsewhere?

All her life, Trisha did whatever she needed to do to survive and succeed. She was optimistic by nature, with a wonderful sense of humor and a ready laugh. When she needed to get a masters degree to teach in New York, she earned one. When her husband's career required multiple transfers during their marriage, she found teaching positions wherever they went. When she needed to have a more flexible career to be there for her young daughters, she harnessed her entrepreneurial spirit and started a home-based marketing business.

And when her husband's constant moves and refusal to deal with his own drinking problem became insurmountable, Trisha concluded that being a single mother was better than the instability of her young family's current life. She made the difficult decision to separate, and eventually divorce.

Even through the difficult times, like the breakup of her marriage, Trisha had always been healthy, energetic and positive. But there was nothing positive about the prognosis of SPTCL. Nothing could have prepared her for this diagnosis.

ARROGANCE AND ITS CONSEQUENCES

Dr. Andrews had said his office would schedule an appointment with the oncologist at once, so she was surprised when they called her back to say the appointment would be ten days away. It would be close to August before she would go to the oncology center in Syracuse.

Waiting for her first oncology appointment, Trisha lived in a strange kind of limbo fluctuating between normalcy, anxiety and resignation. She was frightened about facing her fate. But at the moment she felt normal, not ill or weak, so she continued to golf with her friends, even confiding in them about her diagnosis since some of them were healthcare professionals. Being on the greens gave her mind time to rest from the endless worrying and computer-searches for hope. A doctor who golfed with Trisha thought the diagnosis was odd, and told Trisha she acted too healthy to be suffering from lymphoma.

She thought about the folly of counting calories if her prognosis was so poor, so even with the seriousness of the situation, she found wicked humor and some comfort in the idea that she could go off her diet without guilt. Trisha had no desire to run off to the Bahamas or visit the Far East; she rather liked her life and knew she was doing exactly what she wanted to do, spending time with her family and friends.

Her daughters were so supportive and attentive, stopping by for no reason and talking for hours about nothing and everything. Ashley, who recently finished her psychology degree, tried to ease her mother's anxiety by digging up information on fighting cancer, and supplying books about undergoing chemotherapy.

The day for her first oncology appointment finally arrived. Although she was 52, as she stepped into Dr. Stein's oncology/hematology office Trisha realized she must be the youngest person in the waiting room. For some reason that made her feel both awkward and relieved. She was placed in an examining room, and within a few minutes a man in his sixties with an average build and dark hair entered the room, extending his right hand and introducing himself as Dr. Stein. He held her lab report in his other hand.

"Any chance they might be wrong?" Trisha asked urgently.

To her astonishment, Dr. Stein said he had never before seen or treated this type of lymphoma. He echoed what Dr. Andrews had told her; two independent labs agreed on the diagnosis.

"You'll most likely need aggressive chemotherapy," he advised her, "but in the meantime, I'll be sending you for additional blood work and a CT scan to see if the cancer is spreading." For the first time in over two weeks, she felt a glimmer of hope. Maybe the new tests will show something different, she thought.

In the first week of August, Trisha arrived for her CT scan with eager anticipation instead of dread. She couldn't help thinking they would indicate something new, a better outcome. The imaging technician was very helpful and kept telling her, "I don't see anything." She told Trisha what she was looking for on the scan, showing her the computer monitor and how they look for tumors, while confirming that she did not find any abnormalities. Trisha should have been euphoric, but in the back of her mind she kept thinking—*two independent labs confirmed the results.*

Shortly after the CT scan Trisha remembered something she had felt months before. On her inner thigh was the tiniest lump, deep within the skin. Was this small lump related? She decided she would talk to Dr. Stein about this second lump, get the surgeon to remove it and have it tested as well.

At the appointment with Dr. Stein, she was relieved when he revealed that all her blood test results were normal. He spoke about her seeing a specialist, and then dropped a bomb.

"You'll need to start chemotherapy right away," he announced.

"What you have is very aggressive, and you should understand you better measure your life span in months, not years."

Oddly, Trisha had never considered this would be her treatment option, and certainly not so soon. They wanted to schedule chemotherapy for early September. And she certainly never expected such a grim prognosis. None of this made sense. Her newest tests were normal, she didn't feel sick, and they hadn't evaluated the second lump. This was moving too fast.

Dr. Andrews, her surgeon, agreed to biopsy the second lump. As he excised it, he confirmed that it looked like fatty tissue and did not appear to be unusual. Three days later he called her with the results; it was benign. Again, Trisha dared to feel hopeful. The facts didn't match and she still needed answers, so she made a request to get all of her records. She remembered that Dr. Stein talked about having her first biopsy reviewed by another pathologist, one who specialized in SPTCL. She made the request for him to do that.

Her next appointment with Dr. Stein was coming up quickly, and that would mean facing chemotherapy. She was especially apprehensive because nothing added up, and yet, she wondered if her disease was really as dire as the doctors claimed. What if the lymphoma was spreading and she waited too long for chemotherapy? Dr. Stein had talked with her about CHOP chemotherapy, an aggressive four-week series of three chemotherapy drugs combined with the steroid Prednisone. It was sure to make her extremely sick, and more horrifying, Trisha had read that some people with SPTCL actually died during the chemotherapy administration. She feared that the treatment would be worse than the disease.

Just before the oncology appointment, Dr. Stein's office called to say he was ill and unable to see patients. In his absence his partner, Dr. Spelling, would be covering for him, but the office needed time to sort out the appointments. Trisha hung up the phone and stared at the bare wires and pieces of sheetrock in her kitchen. The unfinished mess and gaping holes of her postponed remodeling project had become a metaphor for the current condition of her life. Nothing fit together and everything was on hold.

Through all of this, Trisha continued to maintain her ties to those around her. She was looking forward to an evening out with her women's executive business club. These women shared the joys and struggles of running businesses, both big and small ones, and the challenges and rewards of life. The group had become a support system as well as a business network. They met periodically for dinner, and this time was special; they were celebrating the successful completion of chemo for one of their members who had been diagnosed with breast cancer. This night they would celebrate life. Trisha still had not told many people outside her family about her situation. Since she was not accustomed to more than an occasional glass of wine, by the time she was on her fourth glass, she was sharing more than she intended.

It slipped out unexpectedly, an explosive personal confession. "I have lymphoma," Trisha admitted. Jaws dropped around the table, and everyone froze in place for that moment. When the moment passed and the hands on the clock started to move again, Trisha found herself surrounded by a dozen pairs of arms all attempting to hug her at one time, well-wishes and affection to hold her up.

Her good friend, Barb, slipped in next to her, and began asking Trisha questions. "Tell me about his. What tests have you had? Who is your oncologist?" She seemed to know just what to ask.

The next day Barb called Trisha and recommended an oncologist, Dr. Kramer, who had treated SPTCL and happened to be a good friend of Barb's. Trisha wasted no time setting up an appointment with him. While waiting to see Dr. Kramer, she received her medical records and began scanning the information and reading the pathology report. So many foreign words, but she was determined to learn the meaning of all the medical terms.

There on the pages of the first pathology report, she saw something no one had told her before. "Suspicious for Subcutaneous Panniculitis-like T-cell Lymphoma," it stated.

"Suspicious!" she shouted out loud. Trisha couldn't believe it. She kept reading.

In the second lab report it said, "Most consistent with Subcutaneous Panniculitis-like T-cell Lymphoma." But the second lab had been told about the first lab's findings and been asked to confirm them. One test followed the findings of the other. In reality, these had not been independent lab tests at all.

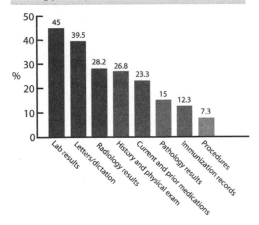

Categories of missing clinical information during primary care visits

Source: Smith PC, Araya-Guerra R, Bublitz C, et al. Missing clinical information during primary care visits. JAMA. 2005; 293: 565-571.

Then she made the most startling discovery. Trisha found the statement, "Specimen being sent for clonality testing." But where were those results? She went to her computer and searched for the word clonality. It meant the replication of cancer cells. There was no report in her records for clonality test results. She called the oncologist's office and told the nurse what she had found. The nurse looked through Trisha's chart, and said how strange it was that the test results on clonality were missing, saying they would have to locate them. Trisha insisted that they send her a copy as soon as the results were located. A few hours later when a fax came through from the medical office, she quickly reviewed the test results. "No clonality present," it read. Trisha was elated.

Several days later, the phone rang and it was Dr. Spelling, the oncologist. "Ms. Torrey, you must start chemotherapy immediately. You have a rare and aggressive form of cancer," he warned her.

Trisha tried to explain to him what she had discovered. "I've been looking over my results. The biopsy was not really from two independent

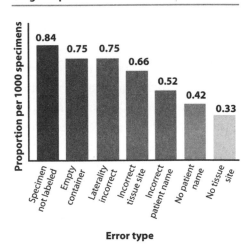

Surgical specimen identification errors

Source: Makary MA, Epstein J, Pronovost PJ, Millman EA, Hartmann EC, Freischlag JA. Surgical speciman identification errors: a new measure of quality in surgical care. Surgery. 2007; 141:450-455. Epub 2007 Jan 24.

labs. My blood work and other tests are normal. This doesn't make sense, and now I have the results of the clonality."

He wasn't listening to her, and he seemed rather annoyed that she would even question his directions. "You have to start chemotherapy, or you'll be dead by Christmas."

"I'm thinking about getting another opinion," she told him.

Dr. Spelling's voice became louder and more insistent. "What you have is so rare, no one will know any more about it than I do, and you're wasting your time," he snapped.

"You arrogant son-of-a-bitch!" Trisha was surprised by the force of her own anger. "I'll find someone else!" She slammed down the phone. She'd had it. They weren't paying attention to the results. She had no symptoms, other than an occasional hot-flash or night sweat, common to every fifty-something woman in the world. Her CT scan was clean, her blood work was normal, her other biopsy benign, and there was no clonality. What game were they playing?

It was September 9, the day of her appointment with Dr. Kramer. He was a quiet, contemplative man in his mid-forties, with a beard and a calm manner. Trisha felt comfortable with him from the moment he entered the room. After her exam, he invited her to his office. He sat behind a big cherry wood desk, holding her lab results in his hand. A large academic textbook that must have contained 2,000 pages rested on

20%

PERCENTAGE OF PATIENTS SEEKING A SECOND OPINION FOR A SERIOUS DIAGNOSIS OR MAJOR SURGERY

his desktop. Dr. Kramer opened it up to *Non-Hodgkin's Lymphoma*, and found the now-familiar words, *Subcutaneous Panniculitis-like T-cell Lymphoma*. It filled less than a third of the page, and said there had been fewer than 100 known cases in the past decade.

Dr. Kramer explained that there were additional diagnostic tests that he could use to confirm or rule out SPTCL, including a bone marrow biopsy and a positron emission tomography, commonly called a PET scan. The scan, he told her, could identify any cancerous areas in the bone, or hot spots, and would show if the cancer had spread. Chemotherapy might not be the option of choice, he said. If other areas of cancer were found on the PET scan, they could be treated with focused radiation.

Listening to this new information, Trisha wondered why this had never been discussed with her before. It was refreshing to have someone give her detailed information and options. She proceeded to tell Dr. Kramer what she had discovered, and how so many things did not coincide with the diagnosis of lymphoma. He listened closely to her and seemed to carefully consider every word. This was the first time during the entire ordeal that Trisha felt she was heard.

"What if I don't have cancer?" Trisha asked him. "You can see all the test results are normal and the clonality is negative."

"You may be right," he answered. His words were a soothing relief that gave her real hope. He said her biopsy could be sent to the National Institutes of Health for additional testing. "I can arrange the NIH testing with Dr. Spelling," he assured her.

12%

PERCENTAGE OF
CANCER DIAGNOSES
THAT MAY BE
ERRONEOUS

On September 20, 2004, three months after that first visit to the doctor, a fax came from Dr. Spelling's office with the NIH results. Trisha fervently searched through the page for the words lymphoma, cancer or malignancy. They weren't there. She quickly faxed the results to Dr. Kramer. He called her the next day to tell her, "You don't have cancer."

"You mean I won't be dead by Christmas?" Trisha asked.

"Start your holiday shopping" Dr. Kramer answered with enthusiasm.

GETTING ANSWERS

Trisha's relief and joy quickly turned to anger. Because of the diagnosis, she had spent weeks of her life believing she was terminally ill with little hope for survival. Although she wrote poignant, articulate letters to both physicians in October, 2004, describing in detail the sequence of events and the misdiagnosis, she never received a call from either Dr. Spelling or Dr. Stein. Her letters also contained direct information from an NIH pathologist, and outlined the poor practices that led to the careless blunder:

- Her benign tumor was ultimately diagnosed as panniculitis, an inflammation of fat cells. The initial testing was wrong, and the suspected diagnosis was not confirmed through the correct channels for rare pathology findings.
- The laboratory testing showed only "suspicious for SPTCL" and "most consistent with SPTCL," and included no follow-up testing.
- A senior pathologist who normally evaluated all rare biopsy results at the laboratory was on vacation in July, when the two analyses of Trisha's specimen occurred. Normally, this pathologist would have reviewed the results and forwarded the specimen to the NIH immediately. Instead, the non-definitive results were returned to the oncologist's office with only suspected findings.

How could two experienced oncologists interpret the lab results without the final pathology report? Why didn't they evaluate all the data, and especially the most significant piece of data related to the clonality? They didn't look at Trisha's clinical picture, including normal test results and lack of symptoms. Neither oncologist closed the loop to confirm the rare diagnosis.

The physicians eventually responded to Trisha in writing, but their letters did not acknowledge the seriousness of what had happened. Likewise, neither one of them took direct and personal responsibility for such a dramatic error. Not only

1/3
Of Survey Respondents

PROPORTION HAVING BEEN A VICTIM OF A PREVENTABLE MEDICAL ERROR WHEN SEEKING CARE

50%
Of Physicians Surveyed

PRACTICING PHYSICIANS ADMITTING TO MAKING A MEDICAL ERROR

did she live through weeks of fear from a false diagnosis, but if she hadn't fought and investigated, she would have received toxic doses of chemotherapy that might have threatened her life or caused permanent damage.

EVERYTHING HAPPENS FOR A REASON

Trisha continues to live a full, healthy life, but this pivotal event changed her forever. "Everything happens for a reason," Trisha says today. She has become an advocate for others, and is leading the way for this new movement. She says, "I am here today advocating for others, an outcome from a horrible experience that can result in good for others." However, that doesn't erase the negative effects of her experience, and even now she continues to suffer from post-traumatic stress syndrome.

She sold her marketing company in the fall of 2006 to begin helping other patients' full time. She built a website full of tools to help those seeking answers, as she once did. Among Trisha's friends her work is known as "Trisha's calling."

There have been other big developments in Trisha's life. Trisha met a wonderful man in February of 2006. They married after dating for a little over three months. "I've never been a person who was afraid to make decisions, and I've never been one to shy away from my intuitive decision-making," she says. "But the one plunge I had never taken was to remarry. One outcome of my misdiagnosis odyssey is that I'm more confident than ever in the decisions I make, and I won't put things off if I know they are important to my happiness."

And Trisha did finish remodeling her house; she made it as beautiful as she felt the day she learned she didn't have cancer.

In healthcare, this type of situation is known as a near-miss; a potentially serious medical error that was caught just in time. A negative cascade of events came very close to causing harm, but disaster was averted through Trisha Torrey's own proactive efforts. She came very close to needlessly undergoing intensive, dangerous treatment, all stemming from a false diagnosis and missing lab results. In other misdiagnoses, a delay in vital treatment can result when the true disease or condition is not properly identified.

There are no exact figures on the prevalence of misdiagnosis, but some statistical and anecdotal evidence shows it may be more pervasive than we realize. Research published in the national publication, *Cancer*, estimates that *nearly 12 percent of cancer diagnoses may be in error*. The study's authors attribute these diagnostic errors to inadequately sampled tissues from biopsy procedures, and recommended using improved methods to detect and correct misdiagnoses.

Studies on misdiagnoses of other diseases and conditions found strikingly similar results to those of cancer. In the July 24, 2003 issue of *The New England Journal of Medicine*, 7,000 medical records from twelve cities were reviewed and revealed that incorrect diagnoses repeatedly led to improper treatments. The study cited evidence that 75 percent of the time, patients with diabetes receive inadequate treatment because of improper diagnoses. The same held true for 40 percent of people with heart disease.

Miscommunication, incomplete paper trails and missing information were found to be major factors in misdiagnoses and improper treatments. Trisha's case was a very real, painful illustration of this problem. Other key issues in diagnostic errors are limited time with patients due to health insurance restraints, and poor follow-up by healthcare professionals.

ERRORS IN DIAGNOSTIC TEST RESULTS

Diagnostic tests can be subject to testing errors, such as inadequate biopsy samples. This can occur if an adequate tissue sample is not obtained, or if the sample areas are not large enough. With any serious diagnosis, such as cancer, a pathology test can be performed at independent laboratories. A patient can request to have their specimen assessed at a different lab with a completely different analysis.

In Trisha's case, the second test was biased because that lab was advised of the first pathology lab's findings, creating a possible preconceived notion about the outcome. A lab can be requested to perform independent or blind tests, not knowing what the first lab concluded. These recommendations should be discussed with the physician so that they can direct the tests.

TYPES OF TESTING ERRORS

Testing errors occur in two ways, known as a false positive or a false negative. This can happen with any test—from a pregnancy test or strep throat culture, to pathology tests for cancer. Trisha's case demonstrated a false positive. False negatives for cancer happen on occasion when an inadequate sample is obtained, or biopsies that return normal later end up showing cancer cells. In either scenario, it is important to seek a second or even third lab analysis to independently test a specimen.

PROTECT YOURSELF IN TODAY'S HEALTHCARE SYSTEM

• Your Right to a Second Opinion—Or Even a Third

System flaws and human errors can still occur, even with the many laboratory quality control measures and regulations. Patients need to be aware of this. For any diagnosis and tests that have serious implications or consequences, such as for cancer or conditions requiring major surgery, a second opinion and second pathology test should be done. Occasionally, even a third opinion or test is warranted.

People should feel comfortable obtaining second opinions on their own, with or without their physician's knowledge. Most insurance companies will cover second opinions for serious diagnoses and procedures. The short period to wait for a repeated diagnostic pathology report, or to see another doctor in a non-emergency, is reasonable.

The American Medical Association encourages the use of second opinions stating, "Physicians should recommend that a patient obtain a second opinion whenever they believe it would be helpful in the care of the patient. When recommending a second opinion, physicians should explain the reasons for the recommendation and inform their patients that they are free to choose a second opinion physician on their own, or with the assistance of the first physician."

There are no widespread studies that can confirm the exact prevalence of misdiagnosis. Nevertheless, misdiagnosis does occur, and a patient should take every step to try and give the physician accurate information about their history and symptoms. People should never hesitate to seek further help from other physicians or sources.

• The Role of Patient Advocacy

Trisha took steps to ensure her own safety. She listened carefully to the physician's evaluation of her diagnosis. But most critically, when other tests didn't confirm a consistent picture of her diagnosis, she began to ask questions. She investigated information from reliable Internet sources, and began reading information that guided her on the appropriate questions to ask. Trisha also paid very close attention to other important test results, such as her blood test, CT scan and her general state of health. Her conclusions were not consistent with what the oncologists told her.

Today there is clearly a shift in how patients are participating in their healthcare. The average consumer now has access to thousands of professional medical websites. They can read about any disease or illness, even the rare ones. Although this does not make them healthcare professionals, people know when something may be wrong with a diagnosis, and they can continue to seek information. This empowerment through information is changing the patient's role in the doctor-patient relationship, with patients taking more responsibility.

There is a growing movement for patient advocacy on a personal level, and through organizations that help patients by providing an advocate or changing policy. People have identified that healthcare is often rushed and the patient is not listened to consistently, and are working to address the issue. Dr. Jerome Groopman, author of *How Doctors Think*, states that on average, a physician has already drawn a conclusion about a patient's symptoms after only 18 seconds.

Trisha's case should not be dismissed as a rare or random occurrence, nor should it indicate that many diagnoses of cancer are wrong. Cancer is a serious and deadly disease that can often be successfully treated when caught early. It is critically important to understand and evaluate a new diagnosis for any type of cancer. But understanding how the diagnosis was obtained is essential. Patients need to thoroughly discuss with their physician the results of cancer pathology tests. There is a need to confirm the specific test results and to assure that all results have been returned to the treating physician for a definitive diagnosis and plan of care.

Seek a SECOND opinion:
- If you are having trouble obtaining a diagnosis.
- If you are diagnosed with a serious illness, such as cancer, or a rare disease.
- If the diagnosing physician is not an expert in the specific disease.
- If you are uncomfortable with the recommended course of treatment.
- If you have been given more than one treatment option for a diagnosis.

Important Points to Remember:
- Talk with your doctor about seeking a second opinion; the AMA encourages physicians to cooperate with patient requests for second opinions.
- Find an expert in the field related to your diagnosis to confirm the condition/disease.
- In most cases, private health plans and Medicare will allow you to obtain a second opinion.
    - Call your health insurance provider or Medicare representative for details.
- If your health insurance provider denies a second opinion, ask for a written explanation. You can appeal the ruling.
- If the first and second opinions differ, Medicare will often allow for a third opinion. If this happen, call you Medicare representative.
- *Important: If a doctor becomes angry, defensive or resistant to your wish for a second opinion, this is a warning sign, and a second opinion definitely should be sought.*

For more information on pathology testing and other topics related to cancer, contact:

- The National Institutes of Health (NIH) Cancer information Service:
  - Toll-free: 1–800–4–CANCER (1–800–422–6237)
  - http://www.cancer.gov/cancertopics/factsheet/Detection/laboratory-tests
- Visit Trisha's Website to inform and empower patients: www.EveryPatientsAdvocate.com
- Visit Trisha's Website with links and resources: www.diagKNOWsis.org

CHAPTER 3

CRITICALLY

In this chapter
- Find out how one medical error can have a domino effect.
- Learn how to prevent hospital acquired infections and what to watch for in the hospital.
- Why should you check the experience and skill level of the surgeon performing a procedure?
- How coordination and sharing of information between all of your doctors is vital to good care.

Why are cascade of multiple medical errors important for you to know about?
In some cases, an incorrectly performed surgical procedure or surgical error can lead to the need for additional procedures and longer hospitalizations. This can increase the risk of hospital acquired infections and open the door to additional serious complications. Piled on top of one another, their effects are magnified on an already weakened body.

WOUNDED

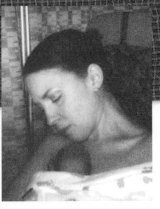

Diana Brookins and baby Julia

At the young age of 25, Diana Brookins was heading her life in a new direction. She was working at a customer service office where she received praise from the managers at her job. In her off-hours she sang and acted. After years of belonging to the church in which her father raised her, Diana began the process of entering into the Catholic Church of her mother's tradition, rediscovering spirituality in her life. She was engaged to be married, and lived in an apartment not far from her mother and step-father. Then in January of 2004, to her surprise, she discovered she was pregnant. Diana knew she and her fiancé were very different people, but trusted that things would somehow work out.

The first person Diana confided in was her mother, Kim. On some level, Diana already sensed that Kim was the one who would ultimately stick by her and be her rock. Kim wanted the best for her daughter, and Diana knew this. It was Kim who was there for Diana's ten-week prenatal appointment at the obstetrician's office, where they listened to the baby's heartbeat for the first time. They both cried when they saw the ultrasound and heard the gentle thumping. The next generation, Kim thought. It was at that appointment when Kim pledged her support to Diana, promising to be there for her and for the baby no matter what happened. Little did she know how this pledge would be tested in the coming months.

Over the past few months, Kim and Diana's relationship had undergone a transformation and they had developed a new closeness. Although Kim had six children, Diana was her only daughter and the eldest of the bunch. Diana had always been spirited and full of talent, with a dancer's agile body and a thick, wavy mane of dark brunette hair. Just like Kim, Diana loved the theatre and music and acted in school and the community theatre. She had a rich, beautiful voice for singing Broadway show-tunes, and Kim's greatest joy was directing her daughter in local drama productions for the small theatre company she and her husband operated. Of all her children, Diana was the one most like Kim. But their mother-daughter relationship wasn't always smooth.

Once upon a time, Diana was wild and rebellious, going through a stage in her early twenties where she drank and partied too much with theatre friends, and followed the wrong people. She developed problems with alcohol that she had to face and move beyond with her family's support. Now Diana's life was on a different course and she felt like everything was coming together at last.

Sunday, April 4, 2004
St. Matthew's Church was packed for the 10:00 A.M. Mass on Palm Sunday. Diana Brookins stood in front of the imposing marble altar with about two dozen other adults, who would be received into the Catholic Church just days later on Easter weekend. The candidates, as they were called, stood in front of the assembled parishioners as they were presented to the congregation. This was the final rite-of-passage before it became official at the Easter Vigil Mass. Each candidate had their sponsor, a Godparent they had chosen themselves, standing with them. Diana had chosen her mother, Kim, as her sponsor, and Kim couldn't have been more touched or proud.

Standing at the altar, each sponsor placed a hand on their candidate's shoulder. As they did this, the priest gave the group a special blessing. Kim felt Diana wince as she touched her shoulder. It was clear she didn't feel very well. After the blessing and a round of welcoming applause from the congregation, the candidates and their sponsors returned to the pews for the remainder of Mass.

The congregation was singing when Kim rushed to follow her daughter down the long aisle and out of the church. Diana had doubled over in pain and then suddenly left the pew. They hurried past parishioners holding hymnals and palm fronds as the two of them made their way to the big, heavy doors at the back.

Outside the entrance to the church, Diana sunk to her knees and collapsed on the cold, wet sidewalk, not bothering to shield her face from the rain. Kim leaned over Diana trying to see what was wrong. Diana curled into the fetal position, clutching her upper abdomen, and tears welled in her eyes as she told her mother how terrible the pain was. People leaving Mass began to gather around them, asking if they could do something to help. Kim accepted help from a couple of onlookers to get Diana to the car, slowly making their way through the drizzle. There was a community hospital not far from the church, located in a sprawling suburb outside of Portland, Oregon.

In the emergency room, Diana informed the nurses she was 16 weeks pregnant. She was so petite and slender, it wasn't immediately obvious. She told them about her problems with gallstones, and that her obstetrician had recommended waiting to have gallbladder surgery until after her baby was born. But he also warned her that if the gallstones grew bigger and blocked the duct going into her gallbladder, they might need to perform emergency surgery.

As they ran tests and evaluated her condition, Diana said she had never experienced pain like this before. The ultrasound showed her gallbladder duct was blocked and she would need surgery. She dreaded the thought of undergoing any procedure while she was carrying her baby, but there was no alternative.

Diana lay on a gurney, staring up at the patterns on the ceiling trying to distract her mind from the pain, and listening to her mother's calming voice. A pretty young woman with shoulder-length blonde hair entered the cubical, and introduced herself as Dr. Davidson. Although the doctor appeared to be barely thirty, she looked tired and drawn. She said she was a surgeon, and explained why they needed to operate soon. Without the surgery Diana could develop serious complications from the blocked duct.

Dr. Davidson said she would be performing a laparoscopic cholecystectomy, a procedure nicknamed a "lap-chole" making a small incision using a lighted scope, in which they would remove the gallbladder. It was a routine procedure, she assured them, and said she recently had done four of them on pregnant women. The baby would be unharmed. If she operated in the morning, Diana could most likely return home that same day, and would quickly recover. The doctor was very confident and made it sound so easy, Kim felt sure it was no big deal. There was never a mention of possible complications or risks.

Monday, April 5

Early Monday morning Diana had her surgery. Kim was waiting for her daughter when she awoke from anesthesia. Considering the circumstances, Diana was doing well and had little pain following the surgery. But as the day passed, her abdominal pain intensified and Kim worried.

Despite Diana's increasing pain, Dr. Davidson seemed to be in a hurry to discharge her and send her home. The nurses taking care of Diana felt she wasn't strong enough to leave the hospital so soon, and advocated for keeping her longer. Dr. Davidson insisted on prescribing Vicodin and sending Diana on her way. One of the nurses stood her ground and convinced the doctor to keep Diana overnight, knowing they could monitor her condition and do a better job of controlling her pain. The additional care during the night seemed to help Diana. They were able to ease her discomfort, and Kim hoped the worst was over as she watched her sleep.

Tuesday, April 6

Dr. Davidson discharged Diana on Tuesday morning, and Kim took her home to the family's contemporary, angular house on the same suburban cul-de-sac where the kids had grown up. Unfortunately, the timing couldn't have been worse for their family.

Kim and her husband, John, needed to make a brief trip that week to Idaho, to pick up their son, Daniel, and take him to his new school in Bend, Oregon. The journey had been planned for weeks. Although she hated to leave, Kim asked Linda, a trusted friend who was a nurse, to stay with Diana while she was away. Kim knew she was leaving her girl in good hands.

Wednesday, April 7

On Wednesday, Kim and John left town to handle the arrangements for their son's school, calling home several times. But by late that evening, Linda told them she was concerned about Diana and thought she wasn't recovering well. She was nauseated. Her abdominal pain continued to increase, despite the Vicodin, and her abdomen was beginning to swell. Linda suggested taking Diana back to the hospital, and Kim agreed that was best. She was anxious to get a quick night's sleep and get back to her daughter by Thursday night.

Kim slept restlessly, and during the night she had a vivid dream about a pregnant woman who died. No dream had ever seemed so real to her. She awakened in a cold sweat feeling panicked, and knew she couldn't wait to drive back with John; she had to get to her daughter as soon as possible. Maybe she was overreacting, but she couldn't shake the feeling. John began dialing the airlines before dawn to arrange a ticket for Kim on the next flight out.

Thursday, April 8

When the plane landed Kim went directly to the hospital from the airport. Walking into Diana's room, she couldn't believe what she saw. Diana's belly was so swollen that she looked nine months pregnant. She was pale, and the heart monitor showed her heart rate was over 100. Kim was shocked at the change. In just two days, Diana appeared to have become alarmingly ill.

"I want to talk to the surgeon now," Kim told the nurse in her most assertive voice.

Dr. Davidson entered the room a short time later, looking calm and unconcerned about the situation. Kim could feel her frustration level rising as she asked about Diana's condition.

"Diana's getting a lot of pain medications, and she's fine," the doctor insisted.

Now Kim felt angry. By the way the doctor said this she was implying that Diana just wanted drugs. Diana's problems with alcohol were part of her medical history, but Dr. Davidson was using that history to make judgments about her current health problems. *How dare this doctor assume my daughter just wants pain medication. Can't she see Diana's in trouble?*

"I want another doctor," Kim said firmly. She sensed this doctor was not someone she wanted near her daughter again.

Dr. Davidson responded that no other surgeons were available.

"Then I want Dr. Wilson, her gastroenterologist. My daughter needs help!" This time Kim was emphatic.

Dr. Davidson left the room without saying a word. Diana told her mother everything that had happened in the last day, and how she was feeling worse by Wednesday night.

At last, Dr. Wilson arrived and examined Diana. He told them he didn't like the look of Diana's abdomen. He wanted to perform a procedure called an ERCP, an endoscopic retrograde cholangio-pancreatography. This would allow him to look through a scope at the biliary ducts and pancreas using a dye. He would be able to see any problems near the surgical area, as well as Diana's liver. By using the scope, Diana could avoid another surgery. He explained that occasionally there can be a leak at the surgical site after an operation. If that was the case, then he would find and treat the area through the scope. Kim felt reassured that Dr. Wilson was here and handling Diana's care. Now things would improve.

They took Diana for the ERCP, while Kim waited for the doctor to report back what he had found. But afterward, the doctor didn't have all the answers as they hoped he would. Dr. Wilson told them he had removed excess fluid and bile from the surgical area, but never explained the source of Diana's worsening symptoms.

Friday, April 9
By Friday night, Diana's pain was so intense that the doctors gave her morphine through a patient-controlled system attached to her IV, called a PCA pump. The nurse explained to Diana and Kim how the pump worked. A computer in the pump supplies a pre-measured dose when the patient feels they need pain medication, and pushes a button allowing it to be released into their IV line. For the first time in over a week, Diana could feel some relief, but her heart continued to race, and her abdomen continued to quickly increase in size.

Saturday, April 10
Despite the morphine pump, Diana's pain intensified. By Saturday, Diana said she wanted to die. Her misery was so horrible she didn't want to go on. The surgeon seemed unconcerned about Diana's pleas, and refused to order additional adjustments to her morphine

dose. Kim felt the surgeon and some of the nurses were ignoring Diana's request, assuming she was seeking a high from the medication instead of trying to escape the unbearable burning and swelling in her abdomen. Both Diana's obstetrician and her gastroenterologist were baffled, and unable to find the cause for her condition. No one seemed to have any answers.

As Saturday stretched into Easter eve, the heart monitor showed Diana still had tachycardia, a racing heart rate. The doctors didn't think they could give her more drugs to relieve the pain. Kim was frightened by Diana's deteriorating condition, and even more by her desire to give up. Diana should have been at St. Matthew's that night, entering the Catholic Church and receiving her First Communion. This should have been a joyful time, but instead they were here and she was suffering.

Kim talked the nurses into bringing a Doppler up to her daughter's hospital room, thinking that the sound of her baby's heartbeat would give Diana the will to live and distract her from the pain. The nurse applied the cold, wet gel to Diana's abdomen and

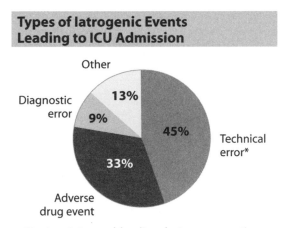

Types of Iatrogenic Events Leading to ICU Admission

Other

Diagnostic error

13%

9%

45%

Technical error*

33%

Adverse drug event

*Such as injury or bleeding during an operation

Source: Lehmann LS, Puopolo AL, Shaykevich S, Brennan TA, Iatrogenic events resulting in intensive care admission: frequency, cause, and disclosure to patients and institutions. Am J Med. 2005; 118:409-413.

gently slid the sensor over her belly. Through the pain, she heard the loud, strong heartbeat of her unborn baby, and Diana drifted off to sleep listening to the rhythmic pulse of new life. On Monday Diana was moved to the intensive care unit.

Monday, April 12

Diana was already thin before her illness, and had been unable to have any nutrition besides her IV solution since she re-entered the hospital before Easter. She was becoming dangerously underweight. The doctors told Kim and her daughter that, for the health of Diana and her baby, they needed to place a PICC line into one of her major veins so they could give her a stronger, more complete nutritional substance. They explained that the PICC line was a peripherally inserted central catheter, like a bigger IV, placed near the entrance of her heart. The solution they would supply through the line was called total parenteral nutrition, or TPN, a mixture of water, glucose, salts, proteins and vitamins. Kim and Diana agreed it was necessary and they inserted the line, but shortly after the procedure the line failed, and they had to perform another PICC line insertion.

Dr. Davidson wanted to put a drain into the abdomen, but Kim and John were so upset by the doctor's management of Diana's care that they begged the nurses not to let the surgeon touch Diana again. The nurses indicated that Davidson was the only surgeon on call, and that her associates were not available to cover for her. As Diana grew worse, Kim had no choice but to let Dr. Davidson put in the drain. She felt helpless and trapped as her daughter still expressed a wish to die because of the unbearable pain.

After the tube was in place, it began draining large amounts of fluid from Diana's abdomen, giving her some relief from the terrible swelling. Dr. Wilson performed another ERCP to relieve additional fluid, but the doctors still couldn't locate the cause of her worsening condition. Kim begged the doctors to do more diagnostic tests, but Dr. Davidson said it looked like Diana was getting better, and the fluid didn't show any signs of infection. For 15 days, the tube never stopped draining fluid.

Monday, April 26

Finally, Dr. Davidson ordered a CT scan, an MRI and a colonoscopy in addition to the ultrasounds. The CT scan revealed a leak from the gallbladder stump where the organ had been removed. The doctor said she and a colleague could perform the surgery to repair the site.

She told them the entire procedure would only take an hour or so.

In the surgical waiting area, Kim and John tried to keep occupied, expecting the doctor to come out any time and tell them it was over and everything was fine. Two hours passed; then three; and no word came. By the fourth hour, Kim was beside herself with worry. A nurse came out and informed them that another surgeon had joined the operation, and someone would come and talk to the family soon.

After eight hours, they saw three surgeons approaching them. They asked Kim and John to come with them into a separate room nearby. Dr. Davidson was there, but sat in a chair and said nothing, neglecting to even make eye contact with anyone. One of the surgeons introduced himself and spoke for the group.

"Diana had a very rough time in surgery. We found a significant leak near her surgical site, and your daughter's intestines are in bad shape. They've been damaged by excess bile in her abdomen," He ended by saying the unthinkable. "We can't promise you another 24 hours."

Dr. Davidson looked down at the floor and remained silent. A shrill cry escaped from Kim, and she buried her head in John's shoulder. John was Diana's stepfather, but he'd grown to love her like his own children. He pulled Kim closer and grabbed her hands, allowing her to lean on him for support.

Kim phoned her sons and her mother, telling them how critically ill Diana had become. They all began making arrangements to fly west and be with her.

Diana remained in the ICU, hooked up to tubes, lines and monitors. It broke Kim's heart to see her, but she felt compelled to be there every moment, keeping a vigil. Diana looked so vulnerable and frail that Kim was afraid she could lose her only daughter, her best friend, the love of her life, at any moment. When Diana regained consciousness, she told Kim she loved her.

Kim was horrified and angered by what this hospital, and especially Dr. Davidson, had done to Diana. She discovered that when they opened up Diana in surgery, part of her intestines fell apart in the surgeon's hands, simply disintegrating. The infection and bile had eaten away her digestive and intestinal tract. There had been a thermal burn from a poorly cauterized gallbladder stump, and a perforation from one of the ERCP procedures. During the surgery Dr. Davidson broke down and had to stop operating. She couldn't function. The staff had to call another surgeon to take over, to help repair Diana's abdomen and intestines.

This hospital had destroyed her daughter's health, and now Kim was done. She wanted Diana moved, transferred to a university hospital in Portland. Dr. Davidson argued, and fought moving Diana. The hospital administration tried to convince Kim to keep her daughter there, but Kim went to the administrators at the hospital in Portland and wouldn't give up. Ironically, a medical professor practicing at the university hospital told Kim that Dr. Davidson had been a fine student. He was surprised to hear of the problems they experienced.

May, 2004

It was a relief when Diana was transferred to Portland, Kim felt more confident about the care she received there, but it was an enormous facility with a maze of corridors going in every direction. They were well into the month of May now, and Diana was making some progress, able to take small amounts of food and regaining some of her strength. She seemed to be healing as the baby grew bigger. An ultrasound revealed that Diana's baby was a girl, and the family felt they had something to celebrate and hang on to. The doctors were optimistic that it might be safe to send Diana home soon, and have a visiting home health nurse to help oversee her care.

During this time, Diana realized that her fiancé was not the person she thought he was, not someone she should share her life with. Because of her illness, she learned she might not ever be able to count on him during the hard times. Breaking off the engagement was painful and difficult, but it was good to find out now instead of later. She would be better off, and so would her baby.

As she healed, Diana was developing a new type of discomfort. She told the doctors and nurses that her chest hurt and she felt like she couldn't breathe well. In response, the hospital sent in psychiatrists to see her and consult with her doctors. Some of them tried to give her medication for depression or other psychological conditions.

Kim found out that Dr. Davidson had continued to call the university hospital long after they had dismissed her from the case, contacting Diana's current physicians and telling them she needed psychiatric evaluation and care. She told them that, in her opinion, Diana's pain was largely in her head. Later Kim would learn that in Diana's medical files Dr. Davidson wrote, *I doubt if this patient's pain will ever fully go away*, implying it existed only in her imagination, despite the serious medical complications Diana had already suffered. Kim was livid. This was a violation of the patient privacy laws, and she confronted the doctors about it, forbidding Dr. Davidson to have any more input on her daughter's care.

They began to prepare the house for Diana's homecoming. Kim transformed one of the boy's old bedrooms for Diana, with a new floral comforter and fresh roses from their garden. John brought in a TV and a small refrigerator so Diana wouldn't have to go far for a beverage or snack. Kim put Diana's knitting supplies by the bed so she could have something to do. She loved to knit and said it relaxed her.

The day arrived when Diana came home, away from the smells and sounds of hospitals, the constant poking and prodding, the unceasing activity and noise. Diana soaked up the peace and quiet, and the way the carpeting muffled sound, unlike the echoing din of the hospital. She reveled in the smells of home, the aroma of cooking and fresh roses and her mother's laundry detergent. The home health nurse showed them how to care for Diana's central line. Kim had lost count of how many central lines Diana had so far—at least a half-dozen. She'd grown to dread the words, "The line is failing and we have to put in a new one."

It was almost two whole days before the pain began again. Diana had become increasingly weak in that brief time. Kim and John took her back to the emergency room at the university hospital, up on a hill overlooking the city. The ER was a busy, formidable place, and they were told Diana would have to be readmitted to the hospital; her central line was failing again. They waited 18 hours, with Diana stuck on a gurney in terrible pain. The staff seemed to be bothered that she wanted more pain medication. She wished they understood what was happening with her body.

Diana told Kim that none of the surgeries or central lines or other problems was as painful as not being believed. It was awful to be trapped in a situation where you couldn't convince anyone that your feelings and symptoms were real.

June, 2004

During the last weeks of May, Kim and John made several unsuccessful attempts to bring Diana home and keep her there, but she was too sick. By early June, the pain in Diana's chest was unbearable, but they continued to treat her as if she was seeking drugs. Kim noticed Diana's color had changed, and she almost appeared to be turning green. A battery of lab tests revealed that Diana had a serious infection in her blood stream, one with a long name: Methicillin-resistant Staphylococcus aureus. They shortened it to MRSA, or mersa, when they referred to it. Diana would need to receive an IV antibiotic called Vancomycin to combat the aggressive staph infection. She was worried about the baby, but they explained the infection threatened them both, and the risk of not treating it far outweighed any concerns about the pregnancy.

An infection control physician treated Diana daily, and they continued to perform tests. But no one seemed to understand the unrelenting pain in her chest. Despite the intensive antibiotic treatments, she became progressively weaker and her blood counts began dropping. The nurses began transfusions of blood platelets to help strengthen Diana and her baby. Her blood pressure became dangerously low. It was clear the MRSA wasn't responding to antibiotics, and the chest pain never subsided.

The doctors confirmed the worst-case scenario; the infection had spread through Diana's blood stream to her heart valve, and she was in septic shock. The echocardiogram showed that her heart valve was damaged. Now her cascade of disastrous medical complications threatened not only the life of her baby, but her own life as well.

July, 2004

Kim was frustrated by the lack of synchronized effort between the medical teams. Because of her multiple medical conditions, Diana had so many different groups of specialists caring for her now: obstetricians, cardiologists, gastroenterologists, infection control specialists. Beyond that, each group of physicians had numerous associates, and most of them saw Diana at one time or another. There was no official central figure coordinating her care and the decisions, making sure everyone had the same information. One physician's assistant tried to help, but it was a tall order for any one person, particularly when they had no authority. To make things more complicated, Kim quickly learned that June is the worst month in a teaching hospital, because of the turnover in rotations for students and residents. Diana was being so brave, knowing that her heart, kidneys and liver were all in danger of failing.

Soon they would have to make a decision about delivering the baby, the doctors said. Diana was now 29 weeks pregnant, and she would need open heart surgery as soon as possible to repair her failed heart valve. The doctors were not sure Diana would survive a Caesarian section, but they weren't confident that she could survive any kind of difficult labor either. Her heart was too weak, and labor was hard work, as the very word implies. They estimated Diana had only a 50 percent chance of surviving a normal vaginal delivery. The doctors decided they would make just one attempt to induce labor, and if it failed, they would have to take the baby by C-section.

In July they chose a day to induce Diana. Female relatives from around the country flew in. Diana's mother, grandmother and some aunts arrived, and the women gathered in the hospital room as the nurses hooked up the oxytocin drip to Diana's IV. They put blankets on the floor as makeshift pallets, and rested while they kept watch, ministering to Diana's needs and lending moral support, the way women did for centuries before doctors and hospitals entered the picture. For hours the nurses monitored her progress hoping to get labor started, but in the end it was unsuccessful. Her body just wasn't ready to give birth in that way, at that time.

On Saturday, July 17, they wheeled Diana toward the operating room. Diana whispered to Kim, voice groggy, "I don't want to die. Pray with me, Mom." Kim fought to keep her composure and be strong for her daughter, but hearing her own baby say she was afraid and knowing she was going in there alone, she felt something break inside her. Diana should never have had to face this, and Kim so wished she could trade places with her. She started to pray the Hail Mary with Diana, and they kept going until the nurses told her she had to leave. Once Diana was safely out of sight, Kim squatted down and leaned back against a wall, crying.

After so many long waits for Diana's other surgeries, they were relieved to have news within minutes. A surgical nurse in green scrubs hurried out of the operating room to the waiting family, and told them Diana had a healthy baby girl. They could see her in the neonatal intensive care unit soon, she told the new grandparents. *Grandparents . . . a baby girl!* For a moment Kim allowed herself the joy and excitement all new grandparents feel, until the realization returned that this wasn't any routine delivery.

Kim stood by the corridor leading to the operating rooms, expecting to see them wheeling Diana out soon after. The thought of what the doctors said about Diana's chances for survival during this delivery was unimaginable. It would be too cruel to have the same day Diana's baby was born, be the very same day Kim lost her own child. Finally word came that Diana was on her way to the cardiac ICU, and the family could see her. She had hemorrhaged from her uterus, Kim was told, but they had stopped it and given her blood transfusions.

Diana looked weak and pale, but peaceful, lying in the ICU cubicle. The burden of worrying about the baby inside her was lifted, and now she could focus on resting and getting well herself. Kim sat in a chair next to the bed and held her daughter's hand. She wanted Diana to know that, even though she loved the new baby, no one could replace the love she had for her only daughter. Leaning close, she whispered into Diana's ear, "You will always be first in my heart." Diana squeezed her hand.

Kim stayed through the night, only leaving to visit the NICU and see Julia Belle. Diana had named her girl in honor of her own grandmother, Julie. The baby was doing well, one huge bright spot in an otherwise bleak summer for their family. She was little, but perfect, and reminded Kim so much of Diana when she was born. Diana had been born prematurely too, and before her birth the doctors hadn't been optimistic about her chances for survival, because Kim had pre-eclampsia. Kim held on to that memory as she sat by baby Julia and touched her feet; stories do have happy endings, she thought.

The next day was Kim's birthday, and her greatest present was Diana's improvement. She lifted her head and told her mother, "I want your world famous potato salad and ribs."

Diana longed to see Julia, and cried because they couldn't be together like other new mothers and babies. The nurses arranged a visit to the NICU, wheeling Diana to the nursery in her hospital bed and pushing her up alongside the baby's warming bed so she could reach out and touch Julia's tiny wrinkled hands and feet.

Although the staff in the NICU was accustomed to private, poignant moments between parents and their tiny, fragile children, this was special. Several nurses gathered around as Diana met her baby girl for the first time. Kim stood nearby snapping photos of the event, finding it hard to focus with tears in her eyes. Like any new mother, Diana wanted to know how much Julia weighed. Two pounds, thirteen ounces, a nurse told her. Diana's eyes leaked a steady, silent stream of tears that dripped down the sides of her face.

"Oh, baby, I can see you are trouble!" Diana said, gently shaking her head, and everyone laughed as their eyes misted.

Over the next few days, Diana seemed to find an inner strength. She knew what she was living for now, and she perked up each time she saw Julia Belle. Diana began eating again. She so badly wanted to leave the hospital. Kim was worried she wasn't strong enough, but Diana fought to go home. She could rest better there, she said, and visit Julia just like she did now, and soon, she would bring her baby home for good.

They were waiting for the heart valve surgery that would restore Diana's health. She was still too weak, the doctors said, and needed to get her strength back before another procedure. After she recovered from the birth, then they could prep her for heart surgery. Six days after the C-section on Wednesday, July 22, the doctors agreed to let Diana go home.

Sunday, three days later, Kim helped Diana slip on a new dress she had picked out for her daughter. She looked beautiful, Kim thought, tired and frail, but so beautiful. They had big plans for the day, and Diana would need all her strength. First they were going out to breakfast, and then up to the hospital NICU to visit Julia.

That morning they had talked about what they would do when Diana was stronger and Julia Belle came home, how she would shop for a blue dress for Julia, and where she would take her for walks. Kim reassured Diana that she could stay at their home as long as she needed, forever if she wanted to.

After they arrived at the hospital, Kim noticed how weak Diana had become. Kim wheeled her to the nursery to see Julia. It would have been too far to walk in her condition. For the first time, they placed the baby on Diana's chest and she held her close, cradling Julia to her body. The baby slept quietly pressed against her skin. Diana closed her eyes and leaned her own face down, resting it on Julia's head, and Kim used her camera to freeze the moment in time. It looked like a perfect portrait of the Madonna and Child. Kim thought she had never seen anything so lovely.

Kim spoke with one of the residents and told him how concerned she was with the way Diana looked. She asked him to admit Diana back into the hospital, but he told Kim that she would have to go through the ER. Diana refused because she remembered lying on a gurney in the ER for 18 hours, waiting for help. She dreaded the thought of returning to that horrible place. Diana kissed her baby goodbye, inhaling her scent before handing her back to a nurse.

At home, Diana told Kim she was tired and wanted to lie down. Kim said she loved her, and left to get the beautiful photo of Diana and Julia printed and framed. It wouldn't take long. She would be back in no time, she told Diana.

When Kim returned, the house was eerily quiet. Something was different. Usually Diana had the TV on for background noise, even when she was sleeping. Kim walked down the hall to Diana's room to show her the picture. She approached the doorway and peered into the room, expecting to see the new dress draped over the chair by the door, but it was empty. As she pushed the door open there was Diana, still in the dress, lying on the bed motionless.

Kim panicked, screaming and crying. She dialed 9-1-1, and then began CPR, all the while praying out loud through her tears, begging for Jesus to raise Diana from the dead like he had done with Lazarus. But it was too late, and Kim knew Diana was gone. Her first-born and best friend had been taken from her, leaving a gaping wound that would never heal.

When she was going about the painful job of planning Diana's funeral, Kim expected a small gathering. She would do the eulogy herself, and she assumed most of the mourners would be family. After all, most of Diana's friends from her school days had moved away and she had led a fairly quiet life in the past few years. But Kim was stunned when over 700 people showed up at St. Matthew's Church for Diana's funeral Mass. It was proof to Kim of how many lives Diana touched.

Kim adopted Julia Belle on the birth certificate, and is now raising her as her own. She wrote a play about her daughter, and hopes that someday Julia will see it, perhaps even perform in it as an actress, just like her mother.

From Palm Sunday, April 4 through Sunday, July 25, 2004, Diana Brookins spent 110 days in the hospital. She was never able to be at home for more than 48 hours at any one given period of time. What was supposed to be a routine, minimally invasive procedure that would require a one-day hospital stay, turned into a cascade of medical errors for this otherwise young, healthy 25-year-old expectant mother and her family.

Diana succumbed to a flood of preventable adverse events that occurred in the hospital. As devastating as one medical error can be to a patient, Diana was inflicted with multiple errors that built one on top of another, none of which were recognized early enough to save her life. Her family discovered later from the autopsy report that the first error occurred during Diana's initial surgery, and the chain of events followed from there.

- The area where the gallbladder was removed had been badly burned at the stump during the initial surgery.
- This injury began the flow of surplus fluid and bile that contributed to Diana's pain as it damaged the surrounding tissues.
- The intensifying pain was not recognized by the surgeon or other professionals as a warning sign of trouble.
- Diana was viewed only as seeking additional pain killers.
- Diana's damaged intestine was perforated during one of the two ERCP procedures she subsequently underwent.
- Both the surgical injury and perforation resulted in the continued abdominal swelling and pain, and the surgical area's failure to heal.
- The excess bile production continued to destroy portions of Diana's intestines.
- Diana was not able to return to normal eating patterns, causing her to need feeding tubes and central IV lines.
- The need for nine central line insertions over the 110 days, and the frequent care to maintain those lines exposed Diana

to invasive procedures that made her vulnerable to the development of a hospital acquired infection.
- Diana contracted an infection within the hospital, from either improper central line insertion or due to careless maintenance of the central lines in place.
- The infection transmitted through one of her central lines went into Diana's bloodstream, causing septicemia.
- Due to Diana's procedure-induced complications and poor nutritional status, she had developed a weakened immune system, rendering her vulnerable to such infections.
- The infection in her bloodstream traveled to her heart, leading to a vegetative (poor functioning) heart valve.
- Due to Diana's weakened condition, damaged heart valve and the delivery of her baby, she did not survive long enough to undergo a heart valve replacement surgery.

5,500

THE DAILY NUMBER OF NEW CASES OF PREVENTABLE HOSPITAL ACQUIRED INFECTIONS (HAI)

$3.5–4.5 Billion

THE EXCESS ANNUAL COST OF CARE FOR PATIENTS WITH HOSPITAL ACQUIRED INFECTIONS (HAI)

The MRSA infection that destroyed Diana's heart valve is a significant and growing cause of adverse events within hospitals in the United States. Healthcare Acquired Infections (HAI) are infections that occur within a hospital, nursing home, or other healthcare facility. HAIs are not related to the original illness or condition. Several types of resistant bacteria cause these deadly infections. These pathogens are grouped into a category called multi-drug resistant organisms (MDRO), including Methicillin-resistant staphylococcus aureus (MRSA), Vancomycin-resistant enterococci (VRE), and certain gram negative bacilli. In addition, there are other strains of resistant organisms that are likely to cause increased resistant infections in the future.

According to the Centers for Disease Control (CDC), the pervasiveness of HAIs in U.S. hospitals is as high as two million infections per year (averaging nearly 5,500 infections per day), and the cost is estimated to be between 3.5 and 4.5 billion dollars in excess cost of care. Widespread over-usage of antibiotics has created mutations of bacteria that no longer respond well to antibiotics.

Staphylococcus aureus is commonly present on people's skin, in the nose and in the environment. In most healthy people the bacteria does not pose a threat to health. However, over the last century, bacteria have become resistant to standard antibiotic treatments, including the penicillin and vancomycin families of drugs. MRSA and VRE infections are continuing to become increasingly resistant to newer antibiotics, and are serious and increasing problems. Within hospitals or other healthcare settings, these pathogens cause severe complications leading to infections of the surgical site, bone, bloodstream and urinary tract, as well as in the lungs, causing a form of pneumonia. Often these infections can destroy multiple human organs, leading to a condition called septic shock, or sepsis. This is what happened to Diana.

In addition to wounds, HAIs can be transmitted through IV lines, catheters, tubes and drains, particularly if these devices are left in the body for prolonged periods of time. Central IV lines are especially vulnerable for originating disease, because these catheters go directly into the blood stream, close to the heart. Usually the lines are used in patients with prolonged illnesses who are unable to take in regular nutrition. These factors often lead to suppressed immune systems.

Infections in central line devices can be relentless and life-threatening. Each year, an estimated 250,000 cases of central line-associated bloodstream infections (BSIs) occur in U.S. hospitals, with an estimated death rate of 12 to 15 percent. The marginal cost to the healthcare system is approximately $25,000 per episode, but some infections can run much higher, into the hundreds of thousands and even millions due to complications and prolonged hospitalization.

PROTECT YOURSELF IN TODAY'S HEALTHCARE SYSTEM

Many HAIs are preventable through excellent hand hygiene. Hand hygiene is defined as the practice of maintaining proper hand cleansing each time a healthcare worker interacts with a patient, including cleaning hands whenever contamination occurs. This can be done through hand washing with soap and water, applying an alcohol-based hand gel and appropriate application of gloves. Hand hygiene is the single most important factor in preventing infections. Nevertheless, data shows that healthcare workers use recommended hand hygiene only 15 to 40 percent of the time. Since MRSA, VRE and other hospital infections are spread through direct contact, this statistic shows frighteningly poor compliance with protocol in preventing infections.

Patients and their families have to be advocates for improving compliance with hand hygiene. When you are first admitted to a hospital, visiting a doctor's office, a clinic or emergency room, tell the healthcare workers that you will be asking them to use proper hand hygiene each time they have contact with you. The following are critical safeguards for patients:

- Upon the first contact with the healthcare professional, set the expectation that you require them to use proper hand hygiene. Remember this can be the use of an alcohol based gel, or hand washing with soap and water.
- Ask the healthcare professional to use hand hygiene each time they care for you.
- Request that healthcare professionals wash their hands before putting on and after removing gloves.
- Ask that a new set of gloves be used each time the healthcare professional cares for you. Healthcare workers often wear gloves from room to room, and this is an unacceptable practice.
- Request that the healthcare professional wash their hands after touching blood, body fluids, secretions, excretions, and contaminated items, whether or not gloves are worn.
- Ask the healthcare professional to wash their hands or use hand gel between tasks and procedures to prevent cross-contamination of different body sites.

Hospital's carry a risk of infection by the very nature of their interactions, including multiple contacts between patients, touching numerous tubing, lines, equipment and surfaces, fast-paced activities and the prevalence of bacteria in hospital units. Cultures taken from different hospital surfaces such as computer key boards, medication carts and table tops have been shown to grow MRSA and other dangerous organisms. It is important to be as diligent as possible to protect yourself or your family member while hospitalized.

If you have an IV, central IV line, catheter, drain or other tubing, ensure that the healthcare professionals use excellent hand hygiene before touching the devices. Ask the nurses how they will be cleaning the devices before giving medications or drawing blood. The ports to these central line catheters should be thoroughly cleaned with alcohol, chlorhexidine or betadine wipes for 15 to 30 seconds. Some hospitals may use other cleaning solutions or a combination of cleaning substances, so be sure to ask what your hospital's policy is, but be certain the policy is followed each time. If a patient is too ill to observe this, then a family member can be an advocate for appropriate line care.

Once you learn the technique and you observe that it is not followed, ask to speak to a nursing supervisor and point out what you have seen. What you do can make a big difference in preventing infections. Patient with weakened immune systems who have central lines are much more vulnerable to infections, although any hospitalized patient is susceptible to a healthcare acquired infection.

At first it may feel uncomfortable to question the practices of healthcare professionals who provide your care, and it may seem tedious to constantly pay attention to the smallest details. But remember, your health and even your life may depend on it.

Help Prevent the Spread of Infections:
- Careful hand washing is important to prevent the spread of infections like MRSA. Ask healthcare professions to wash their hands or use antibacterial hand gel each time they care for you.
- If a healthcare professional appears frustrated or defensive when you ask them to wash their hands, keep insisting that they use proper hand hygiene. This is for their protection as well as yours.
- The spread of infections can occur through improper cleaning of devices. Ask the nurse how the IV ports or catheters are cleaned.
- Multi-Drug Resistant Organisms (MDROs) can be spread through close contact with someone who is carrying the bacteria, especially by the hands or contaminated gloves, as well as by other exposed items. It is not spread through the air. Proper hand hygiene is essential.

Isolation Precautions:
- Actions to prevent the spread of harmful germs from one patient to another are called isolation precautions.
- The precautions used depend on the type of microorganism.
- If someone in your family is in isolation, a nurse should explain the type of isolation precautions necessary.
- Read and follow any instructions carefully.

Resources For You:
- Information about MRSA in the healthcare setting can be found on the CDC webpage for Antimicrobial Resistance

CHAPTER 4

PICKING UP THE

In this chapter
- Learn about the safe use and potential dangers of patient controlled analgesic (PCA) pumps for post-surgical pain medication.
- Why you should find out before surgery how your hospital monitors patients on intravenous pain medication.
- Find out why you should make sure your hospital stocks Narcan on their post-operative unit.
- See a list of recalled PCA pumps that can be dangerous.

Why are errors associated with IV pain medication important for you to know about?
Hospitals use infusion pumps and patient controlled analgesic pumps to administer drugs to patients, most often narcotic pain medications after surgery. In most cases these pumps are safe and effective, but malfunctioning or misused pumps can result in permanent injury or death from an overdose.

PIECES

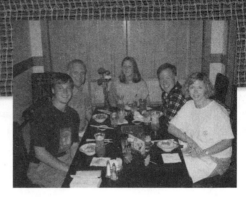

The Ford Family

Dan Ford stood at a podium on the dais, in front of the large crowd there to attend a patient safety conference. His mouth was dry from nerves and anticipation, and he was grateful for the glass of water someone thought to place within easy reach. In his professional work he was accustomed to speaking in front of people but it was different when he was talking about his personal life. Although he had given this presentation nearly 30 times before, it was never easy. While sharing his personal experience was rewarding, and he hoped useful, revisiting the past and laying himself bare could also leave him somewhat drained. But he felt compelled to do it.

As he began to speak he looked out on the chairs arranged in neat rows, filled by healthcare professionals and risk managers who had come to listen and learn. This two-day conference in Las Vegas was dedicated to teaching professionals in the healthcare industry how to improve patient safety using data, prevent medical errors, and improve their response toward patients and their families when things go wrong. This was Dan's passion now. It gave some purpose and meaning to what he and his family had gone through. And like a virtual time machine, the spoken words of his own story transported him back to May of 1991.

Diane and Dan Ford lived in a western suburb of Chicago with their three children, Sarah, age 11, and teenaged sons Jonathan and Chris. Dan worked in the healthcare industry, doing executive recruiting for hospital administration positions. Diane was a trim, attractive woman with blonde hair and brilliant blue eyes, and as a young woman had worked as a flight attendant for PanAm. She was bright as well as pretty, with a master's degree in education, and now she was earning a second master's in theology while running the house and raising the kids. They were the quintessential middle-class family, successful and involved, active in their church and local schools. They were the kind of family many people look at and want to emulate. But the hum of their ordinary-yet-blessed life stopped abruptly one day, permanently shifting the axis of their world.

Like many women in their late forties, Diane suffered from uterine fibroids that caused severe pain and frequent heavy, unexpected bleeding. After years of debilitating symptoms, her gynecologist recommended a hysterectomy to end the problem once and for all. It would be a routine procedure, one of the most commonly-performed surgeries in America.

The gynecologist admitted Diane to the local community hospital. Dan had complete confidence in the facility. After all, it was located in an affluent suburban area that attracted quality physicians and staff. It must be a good hospital, certainly more than sufficient for such a routine matter.

Waiting for Diane's hysterectomy to be over, Dan wondered why it seemed to be taking so much longer than expected. He was getting concerned when, finally, Diane's gynecologist and the surgeon came out to speak with him. Her colon had been nicked during the surgery, they said, and it had required immediate attention to repair it. They had to perform a temporary colostomy, bypassing the colon, and for the next several weeks her bowel would be connected to an opening in her abdominal wall with a bag to collect waste.

Dan was upset by the complication, but relieved his wife would be alright. This meant Diane would be in the hospital a bit longer, and she would likely be in more pain. At least the doctors had recognized the problem and were able to fix it quickly. When she was settled in a hospital room, he went to sit with her. She was still groggy. Dan tried to explain to Diane about the complication and the need for the colostomy. Diane seemed to comprehend what Dan was saying, nonetheless she was astounded at hearing this and then drifted back to sleep from the lingering effects of the anesthetic. The nurses spoke with Dan as he was preparing to leave, assuring him that Diane's post-operative pain would be controlled with the PCA pump (patient-controlled analgesic) connected to her IV line. Whenever Diane began to feel pain from the surgery, she could press the button on the PCA pump to administer morphine (a narcotic analgesic), and keep on top of the discomfort before it became overwhelming. Knowing all this and with Diane resting comfortably, Dan went home to see his family and get some sleep.

Twelve hours later Chris stumbled to the phone, attempting to stop the ringing before it woke everyone in the house. He was up late working on a paper for school. When he picked up, the nurse was on the other end, calling to tell them something had gone wrong. There had been a problem. Please come to the hospital. Chris quickly woke up his father. The drive to the hospital was a blur to Dan. He wasn't sure how he even got there or what route he took.

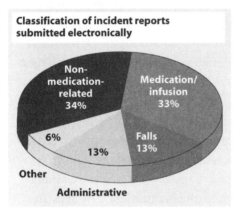

Classification of incident reports submitted electronically

Source: Milch CE, Salem DN, Pauker SG, Lundquist TG, Kumar S, Chen J. Voluntary electronic reporting of medical errors and adverse events. J Gen Intern Med. 2006; 165-170. Epub 2005 Dec 22

After seeing the state Diane was in, he began to ask questions about what had happened. The answers were confusing. Apparently, a student nurse walking by Diane's room late that night had heard her making a strange, abnormal snoring sound, and found her unconscious. The code team was called immediately, but it took another 21 minutes to begin delivering oxygen to Diane's lungs.

A doctor had trouble inserting the breathing tube, and didn't have medication which would have relaxed her throat and made the insertion easier. To make matters worse, no Narcan was available in the unit, a drug that counteracts the effects of narcotic overdose when it's promptly given to patients. By the time Dan arrived, the PCA pump had already been hastily removed and the tubing thrown away. Diane was still unconscious.

Dan traveled back home to tell the kids. They were supposed to go to school that day, but they insisted on returning to the hospital to see Diane. Sarah wanted her mother. When she arrived at the hospital, she sat by the head of Diane's bed for hours and talked to her, stroking her hair. Diane remained in a coma for another 15 hours with Sarah by her side. When Diane eventually awoke late that day, life was unalterably changed for everyone.

Diane wondered what was wrong and couldn't understand what had happened to her. She had no recollection of the colostomy, and didn't know why she had a bag attached to her. The nurses told Dan she might have some temporary short-term memory loss from the oxygen deprivation. Working in the healthcare industry, Dan believed in the healthcare system. He was hopeful about his wife's recovery.

After a couple of days passed, it became clear Diane's problems were more severe than anyone had indicated. She kept repeating the same questions over and over. He had the feeling that nobody in the hospital knew what they were doing, and they were as unprepared as he was to deal with this untoward situation. In hindsight, Dan wished they had gone to a teaching hospital for the surgery, somewhere larger and better equipped.

The doctors said they were optimistic that things might get better, that there might be some re-growth of her brain synapses. In the meantime, the hospital staff and her family began using the whiteboard in Diane's room as a tool to help her remember information. She could look at the board instead of constantly asking questions. Dan noticed some slight improvement in the first days after the coma, but then she seemed to stop making any further progress.

Little help was offered to Dan and the family to help them cope. He felt like a deer caught in the headlights of a car, completely stunned and taken by surprise, with no idea about how to proceed with their lives. There was no coordinator or social worker to assist him with finding the resources they would need. A colostomy nurse in the hospital tried to help, and talked to Dan about some of what he could expect. The nurse seemed to understand the impact of Diane's memory loss. She attempted to teach Diane how to care for her colostomy bag, but Diane had trouble even remembering she had a bag, or why it was there. Eventually she was able to at least drain the bag, but never learned how to change it. It became a constant indicator of the extent of her memory loss.

The day before Diane's release from the hospital, she was

evaluated by a psychiatrist, but it didn't yield any new insights or lead to any additional help. Dan took her home to her family. They brought up a big whiteboard they had sitting in the basement, and placed it in the bedroom so Diane could refer to it often. Daytimers became essential to Diane's ability to function. She could see at a glance what was happening each day from hour to hour, or what she should be doing. Several weeks after leaving the hospital, Diane was seen by a psychologist, but to no avail. It was becoming clear that the damage was physical and the amount of healing would be uncertain.

Their housekeeper, who had worked for them before the surgery, took on new duties helping with Diane's care. Members of their church worked out a schedule to be there when Dan had to be gone for work or business trips, and they helped with meals and errands. A nearby neighbor and Dan's sister became a godsend, checking on the kids and assisting with transportation.

At the end of Diane's first week at home, their son Chris had to have orthopedic surgery on his ankle. Two weeks later, he hobbled across a stage on crutches to receive his high school diploma. At a time in his life when he needed mom's help, praise and attention most, the family dynamics had shifted dramatically. A role reversal had occurred, and now the children were parenting Diane.

While it was terrible that Diane had lost her analytical skills and memory, her mental disability was not the most devastating problem. Overnight, Diane's personality had completely changed. She had been transformed from a mature, loving, caring individual, into someone who was bitter, hostile and frequently verbally abusive. Her emotions reverted to those of a young teenager and she became self-centered, lacking internal controls. She would say horrific things to Dan and some times to her family, vicious words dripping with resentment and sarcasm. Everyone around Diane was constantly on the defensive, afraid of her next tirade or painful comments. Many of these words became increasingly targeted at Dan. He and the children were hurt and confused by her behavior. Dan prayed daily that the kids wouldn't wake up with serious emotional problems ten years down the road. Diane was lost in a shell of what she had been and none the fault of her own, but a preventable medical error that should never have happened.

Two months after her hysterectomy and colostomy, Diane underwent another surgery to reverse the colostomy and get rid of the bag. Just weeks after the reversal surgery, Diane awoke with pain from a kinked colon, an unfortunate residual of her reversal surgery. She was in great discomfort. Fortunately, no surgery was required, but she spent five rough days in the hospital, continually drinking a horrible liquid that kept her intestines empty. Her kinked colon resumed its normal shape, relieving the discomfort. However, a couple of weeks later she discovered something wrong. An examination revealed that a fistula had formed during the reversal surgery healing process and a loop of bowel had broke through into her vagina, an unintended connection between two organs,

Not wanting to put Diane through yet another surgery, doctors waited several weeks to see if the fistula would heal on its own, but it didn't improve. This meant one more surgery three months later, in November, to repair the fistula. When they opened Diane's abdomen, they found stray staples from the colostomy reversal that had migrated from where they belonged, and caused internal damage. These wounds led to the formation of the fistula. They were able to remove additional staples that had broken loose and could cause even more damage.

While trying to deal with the chaos of their family life and trying to handle his work life, Dan began to ask pointed questions of the hospital. At first the exchanges were polite. He asked to see Diane's records, and tried to find out what had occurred on that night of the first surgery. Dan was able to get Diane's hospital records, but Dan's requests to get copies of committee meetings where Diane's case had been discussed fell on deaf ears. He was told these documents were protected under law and he had no right to see them. Following this, the hospital administration became more and more difficult to deal with and defensive.

Conversations with the hospital's risk manager became increasingly strained, as Dan was met with roadblocks and avoidance. The inhuman treatment by the risk manager was offensive. He seemed immune and non-caring to the significant quality of life changes experienced by Diane and the terrible impact on the Ford family. He seemed to have no motivation to be fair to Diane and her family. Dan was treated like a nuisance. The medical errors had happened under the responsibility of the providers, who accepted no accountability for what happened to Diane. The risk manager told Dan that his job was to save the hospital money, period, and he was combative when they spoke to one another. Dan wondered why the hospital didn't have Narcan available, since at the time of Diane's surgery the drug had been a recommended, routinely stocked drug in all hospitals for over a decade. And what had caused the overdose? Did the pump malfunction? There were attempts to explain to him, which seemed like obfuscation at the time. Dan couldn't get answers.

At home, Diane continued to make life emotionally painful for the members of her family. She was suspicious of some around her, and accused them of things they hadn't done. The number of friends she had gradually dwindled, mostly because of her disability, sometimes because of her constant "woe is me" behavior. She complained and criticized constantly, and drove away some of the very people who had wanted to help her.

Dan felt he was at the breaking point. He tried desperately to talk to Diane about his feelings, but she didn't seem capable of caring about anyone else anymore. As a Christian and an active member of his church, Dan took his marriage vows seriously. But he didn't know how to keep doing what he was doing, living in the middle of the madness, trying to stay sane.

Four years after the medical error that had destroyed their former lives, Dan moved into an apartment near their house, where he could still keep an eye on Diane and help care for her. After continued efforts to make Diane's life better and still being seriously criticized too many times by her, Dan thought he was going down the tubes and might not make it. He felt pulled in two opposite directions by his ideal image of what a responsible husband was on the one hand, and by his desperate need to preserve his sanity and health on the other. He was honest with the kids, but they were upset and torn. His moving out had more to do with her significant personality change than her disability, though it compounded it. The kids would still be able to see their Dad when they liked. Diane continued to live in the house, trying to be independent. She received some organized assistance from specially-trained members of their church, who participated in a Stephen Ministry program. They helped those with serious issues, including disabilities. However, any independence was elusive with her memory and judgment severely affected.

A few months after Dan moved into the nearby apartment, a friend of Diane's convinced her to file for a divorce from Dan and to his surprise, she did. With the kids grown, Dan reluctantly began talking with a half-dozen acquaintances he knew professionally who had lived through tough marital situations following a serious illness or injury of a spouse. These individuals were principled, religious people, and yet they had left their marriages when things became hopeless. How were they able to reconcile their faith and moral values with their emotional survival and well-being, he wondered? He never thought this would happen, but he felt he had nothing left to give and allowed the divorce to proceed.

Diane could no longer prepare a meal or read a book. If she went to a movie and had to go to the restroom, she couldn't remember where her seat was and would become lost. If someone asked Diane what she ate for breakfast, she was unable to tell them. She tried to drive, but was too slow and became confused. One day, she went to Nordstrom and bought more than $9,000 worth of clothes in one shopping trip, and Dan had to intervene with the store when the bill came. Her condition was much like someone with Alzheimer's disease, but without the physical deterioration.

Almost two years into their ordeal, the hospital offered a small financial settlement. It was the equivalent of what a legal defense would cost. "It was an insult," Dan now says. Diane's short-term memory and ability to learn were permanently destroyed, and she could no longer earn a living or take care of herself. Their finances were stretched and their lives were in shambles. They turned down the offer. After trying for 21 months to reach a resolution with the hospital and Diane's healthcare providers, Dan and Diane filed a lawsuit.

For the next few years, Diane lived in the same community, with help from her family, church members and other friends. Dan supported her financially, through divorce alimony maintenance. Eventually Diane's brother in Tennessee invited her to come and live there, in an independent living facility. He took responsibility for

Diane and managed her money, placing her on a budget in an attempt to control her indiscriminate spending. Still suspicious, difficult to get along with, and with frequent arguments about money management, Diane became very critical and they had a serious falling out. It was clear she had a need to continue to be in an independent living facility, where trained professionals could provide practical help and support, but she could have some degree of personal independence. Her brother had a Tennessee court appoint a legal Conservator. Diane and Dan's son, Chris, took on these responsibilities and moved her to an independent living facility in Michigan where she continues to reside.

Dan moved to Arizona to make a fresh start. He continued pushing forward with the lawsuit, but it seemed to go nowhere for over nine years. After endless times of dealing with attorneys, Diane lost interest in the lawsuit and basically quit. All she wanted was a functioning brain. The plaintiff's attorneys went back to the hospital attorneys and a minimal settlement was reached in 2002. The hospital's and physicians' legal strategy had worked, dragging out details that wore Diane down, taxing her short term memory and confusion. The spirit of medicine and healing seemed irrevocably violated by this insulating display of legal pandering.

The fact that Dan worked in the healthcare field had not given them any advantage in getting answers or justice, he felt the opposite had happened. Because he was an industry insider, hospital administrators and healthcare professionals seemed to adopt an attitude of knowing indifference toward Dan's plight. Since Dan worked in the business, he should know how things are done. They figured Dan, above all people, should understand there would be no open disclosure. Secrets must be kept. Dan felt their concerns were dismissed because he worked in the system.

It was especially frustrating to be excluded from the reviews of Diane's case. The hospital conducted peer review, but that dealt with the healthcare professionals and was considered a private personnel matter. Dan could have no input, and would never know the committee's findings or what consequences there were for those involved. Dan felt people ought to be able to share their experience with these committees and obtain some information, because after all, it's their bodies at the center of these cases.

Dan knew he wanted to do something to help facilitate change in the healthcare system. "Most people don't want to sue," he says now. "You hit a bump, an error, and suddenly a wall of silence goes up between the patient and the medical professionals and this is human nature. However, everything the providers and their attorneys do after that determines if the wall disappears, stays the same or becomes higher and thicker. Silence or condescending behavior causes speculation and anger which fuels more negative feelings and often can lead to lawsuits. Healthcare professionals don't understand that the relationship determines what happens."

Needing a change in corporate culture, Dan resigned in August of 2002 from the healthcare executive search firm of which he was one of the founders and a major shareholder. He also wanted the flexibility to become actively involved as a volunteer in consumer patient safety. He works with the Furst Group in Arizona. The company better fits his values and sensibilities about the healthcare industry. He brought his passion for patient advocacy to his work, filling positions by now recruiting healthcare executives and outside directors of Governing Boards who share his concerns about and passion for patient safety.

A woman who became the Executive Director of the National Patient Safety Foundation invited him to join a special committee on patient safety of the American Society for Healthcare Risk Management (ASHRM) and talked him into speaking about his experiences. This led to speaking engagements at provider medical and patient safety conferences across the country and an international conference. Speaking on safety led to an even greater involvement for Dan. He was asked to join committees in several organizations that deal with patient safety, quality and patient and family-centered care, including the Institute for Healthcare Improvement (IHI), the Joint Commission, the Arizona Hospital and Healthcare Association (AzHHA), Carondelet Health Network in Tucson, Arizona and Catholic Health Partners in Cincinnati, Ohio.

Diane resides in an independent living facility in Michigan, and her oldest son, Chris, lives close by with his wife and children. She leads a relatively simple life. Once a week Chris takes her to get her hair and nails done, and they run errands together. Dan continues his strong commitment to improve patient safety. Dan's interest and primary focus are to plant seeds of constructive change. He feels one way he can continue to honor Diane and her struggle is to tell their story, and to keep working to improve patient safety in an effort to prevent future medical errors like the one Diane suffered.

Dan has never been able to achieve some measure of closure with the hospital. After repeatedly trying to contact them over the past several years, he still has not received any response or answers, even though the statute of limitations and his acceptance of the settlement mean there is no longer any action he could take against them.

Nothing can restore Diane Ford to her former self, or restore the wife and mother Dan and his three children once knew. But through this event that never should have occurred, Dan has been able to shine a light on a part of healthcare that was traditionally kept hidden from view, swept out of sight before it could be examined. By bringing medical errors out of the shadows and illuminating them, patients and healthcare professionals stand a better chance of fixing a system in distress.

More than 200,000 hysterectomies are performed each year in the United States, and most result in successful recoveries and outcomes. However, Diane's routine hysterectomy was complicated by an error in surgery. *Fireballs* is a term sometimes utilized to describe benign fibroids in the uterus. Fibroids affect tens of thousands of women, and as the nickname suggests, they can be torturous, producing severe pain and abnormal bleeding. Diane suffered from abnormal bleeding for years, and because she had already given birth to three children and was 47 years old, the treatment of choice was to remove her uterus. When the surgeon was removing Diane's uterus, he nicked her colon. The injury was significant enough to require immediate repair, and a colostomy was performed. A colostomy connects a portion of the colon with the abdominal wall, leaving an opening to the outside of the body. This opening is fitted with a seal, and a bag into which the body waste empties. A colostomy is done when the colon must be bypassed for rest and repair, because of an illness like cancer, or due to an injury or trauma. Depending on the type of injury or illness, the colostomy can be temporary or permanent. Diane's colostomy was expected to be temporary, and most likely she would have successfully recovered from her hysterectomy and colon repair within two months. Instead, a very different outcome occurred.

Patient-controlled analgesia (PCA) or infusion pumps are designed to provide patients with pain control for an illness or injury, and they are frequently used after surgical procedures. Many manufacturers produce infusion pumps and, over the last three decades, multiple models have been created.

The pumps are usually loaded with a prescription opiate, such as morphine or dilaudid. Time and amount limits are programmed into the PCA pump, to allow the patient to infuse the needed amount of pain medication, while protecting against accidental overdose. Safety features are included, such as locking key pads to avoid accidental programming errors. Even so, a variety of errors have occurred with PCA pumps, such as equipment failures, electrical problems, medication dosing errors and operator errors.

There was speculation that Diane's over-sedation might have been related to a pump tubing problem, however the exact cause was never revealed to her family. Diane's breathing problems were discovered accidentally by a student nurse passing by Diane's room, so it was never known how long Diane was having problems before she went into respiratory arrest. Once the student nurse sounded the alarm, a code team was called to Diane's room, and the fatal sequence continued.

- No heart or breathing alarm was present to warn the nurses that Diane was not breathing.
- Although the code team was called, the code physician could not readily place the endotracheal tube (breathing tube) in Diane's airway.
- The code team did not have the proper medication to relax Diane's airway to facilitate the tube insertion.
- It took 21 minutes to put the breathing tube in place.
- The code team did not have the drug Narcan available to reverse the effects of an opiate medication, which helps a person to breathe spontaneously.
- Diane suffered irreversible brain damage from the delayed oxygenation.

Top seven barriers to implementing patient safety systems

1 | Competing priorities for scarce resources in a system where patient safety is not considered a top priority.

2 | Lack of resources: inadequate staffing and work overloads.

3 | Availability and cost of patient safety technology.

4 | Resistance to change (the assumption that providers are already providing safe care).

5 | Culture of blame (current healthcare culture is punitive in nature).

6 | Lack of senior leadership understanding of and involvement with patient safety issues.

7 | Culture of healthcare workforce perceptions, attitudes and behaviors of error "cover up."

Source: Barriers to implementation of patient safety systems in healthcare institutions: leadership and policy implications. Akins RB, Cole BR. J Patient Saf. 2005; I:9-16.

Diane's delay of intubation - the breathing tube placement - also may have been caused by a lack of skill on the part of the physician who was performing the procedure.

Narcan was approved by the FDA on April 13, 1971, and widely distributed to hospitals in 1974. It has been used routinely within hospitals by emergency personnel and paramedics in the field to treat overdoses of narcotics. Narcan blocks the opiate receptors in the brain and allows for the return of normal respiration. For many years, it has been a standard drug on hospital crash carts that are utilized for respiratory and cardiac arrests.

Needless to say, there were many fatal points along the way where preventative measures would have avoided this catastrophic medical error. As reviewed in earlier chapters, often when the first medical error occurs, a cascade of adverse events follows, each one leading to the next. The damage to Diane's colon no doubt caused the need for additional pain medication. A routine hysterectomy requires appropriate pain management after the procedure, but with the additional damage to the colon and creation of the abdominal opening for the colostomy, it is likely more pain medication was required. Because of the increased narcotics, heart and respiratory monitors should have been used.

The night Diane stopped breathing was her first night following surgery, when the pain would have been the most intense, and she would need higher doses of morphine. Monitoring during this time may have prevented a full respiratory arrest. In addition, a crash code cart that had the appropriate emergency drugs may have led to a significantly different outcome for Diane.

PROTECT YOURSELF IN TODAY'S HEALTHCARE SYSTEM

There are many critical safeguards to consider when recovering from surgery and utilizing a PCA pump. Human error is the first and most important thing to be aware of when a PCA pump is in use. Request the following information:

- Ask for complete instructions about the use of your particular model of PCA pump prior to operating it.

- Learn what medication and dose you will be given.
- Report all allergies to everyone giving you medication in your pump, especially if you are allergic or sensitive to narcotics.
- Ask the nurses caring for you how much experience they have had with PCA pumps.
- Request to have nurses who have utilized PCA pumps multiple times, and who can demonstrate to you a clear understanding of the use of PCA pumps and their safety features.
- Insist that two experienced nurse's double check the dosage, programming and equipment of your PCA pump.
- Consider asking a pharmacist to review the dose of medication loaded into your pump.
- Insist that you be the only one to use the pump and controls. Patients are the only ones that should deliver a dose of pain medication via the PCA pump controls. Adverse events have occurred when patients ask nurses or family members to administer medication through the pump. When a patient is alert enough to administer more pain medication, there is less chance for over-sedation. If the patient is too sleepy to administer more narcotic infusions, then this is a natural safety sign that appropriate pain relief has been accomplished.
- Tell your family and visitors they should not touch or push the PCA buttons, even if you ask. When other people administer the medication at the patient's request, especially if the patient is groggy or sleepy, then there is a higher risk that another person will administer too much medication. This is called "PCA by proxy," and is a dangerous practice.
- Ask that warning labels be placed on the pump controls stating that only the patient administer the PCA doses. The labels should say, "For patient use only," on the buttons or equipment.
- Remind visitors to contact the nurse if they have any questions about the PCA pump.
- Tell family and visitors to notify a nurse if you seem overly sleepy or hard to arouse.

MORE ON PCA BY PROXY

An incident published by the Institute for Safe Medication Practices described a case where a 72-year-old woman underwent cancer surgery and her surgeon prescribed a PCA pump with a morphine 2 mg loading dose and 1 mg every 10 minutes as needed for pain. The maximum dose was 6 mg-per-hour.

Initially the patient was restless and agitated in the post-anesthesia care unit. Because of this agitation, the nurses interpreted this as a response to pain, despite the patient's inability to verbalize what she was feeling. Nurses pushed the PCA button and delivered frequent doses of morphine over the next 48 hours. Subsequently, the patient suffered a respiratory arrest and seizure, leading to hypoxic brain death, or brain-death from oxygen deprivation. The woman died several months later without ever regaining consciousness.

PCA PUMP EQUIPMENT

Equipment issues are another concern with PCA pumps. Since the inception of the pumps, multiple equipment flaws have occurred causing FDA recalls (see safety keys for the details of those recalls). PCA pumps should never have a system that allows for a free flow of solution into a patient. When patients administer doses of medication, they should be able to both hear and see a confirmation of the dose they receive. Otherwise, the patient may be tempted to keep trying to administer the medication, not realizing the dose was successfully infused. Manufacturers should provide a patient-friendly guide for use of the pump. These instructions should be simple and clear, with appropriate diagrams.

EMERGENCY REVERSAL DRUGS

Narcan should be readily available on hospital units whenever narcotics are used in PCA pumps. This can be stored in the medication area, in an automated dispensing medication cabinet or on a unit's crash cart. A patient can ask the nurse where the Narcan is located on the unit, and how readily it can be accessed.

All nurses on the unit should be familiar with Narcan and its use. In the event of over-sedation from a narcotic, Narcan can be injected into the IV port that the PCA pump utilizes. In the event of an over-sedated patient, the narcotic dosage should be immediately stopped and evaluated by a physician, pharmacist or nurse. The narcotic dose may need to be decreased after an event, and the equipment and pumps should be rechecked for accuracy.

CHANGES IN INFUSION PUMPS

Hospitals have dealt with serious adverse events from infusion pumps in the past. Because of regulatory requirements, earlier model pumps have been replaced with pumps that have advanced safety features. In 2003, the Joint Commission, the organization that accredits hospitals and healthcare facilities, required hospitals to eliminate all IV and infusion pumps that allowed for a free flow of medications.

Newer models have safety tubing and safety mechanisms within the pump that prevent the free flow of the infusion solution. *Smart pump* is the term used to describe new technology to prevent programming errors and free flow. These pumps are considered to have a "test of reasonableness" to check that programming is within pre-established institutional limits before infusion can begin. However, the use of smart pumps is a new technology, and caution should be taken to recognize that problems still can occur even with improved products.

Many hospitals have completed extensive evaluations of their infusion pumps using a process called failure modes and effect analysis, or FMEA. This is an elaborate process that assesses all potential danger points, and builds in safety steps to prevent failure points and errors. In addition, most facilities have developed clear and concise policies and protocols on the use of PCA pumps. Some hospitals only use one or two models and provide competency checks for all personnel using these pumps.

Because there are many manufacturers and models of infusion pumps, little standardization exists across U.S. hospitals. Several cities have multi-hospital patient safety consortiums that work to establish similar practices among local hospitals. But standardized practices are very limited, and are in the early stages of development. Even with protocols or standardized practices, there is no guarantee that fail-proof systems are in place for all of these devices.

NOT FAR ENOUGH

Even though Diane Ford's medical error occurred in 1991, by 2003 the Institute for Safe Medication Practices (ISMP) continued to report multiple errors with PCA pumps. In a paper published by the ISMP, called *Pain Control in Hospitals Using PCA Pumps Must Be Made Safer,* Michael Cohen, ISMP President and founder, stated that these pump errors are preventable through basic actions taken by U.S. hospitals. The ISMP suggests the following recommendations for hospitals:

- Establish selection criteria for PCA pumps. Use the right pump for the right patient.
- Develop protocols and standardized order sets to guide the selection of drugs, dosing, lockout periods and infusion devices.
- Carefully monitor patients. Opiates, even at therapeutic doses, can suppress respiration, heart rate and blood pressure, so the need to monitor and observe cannot be overemphasized.
- Require two clinicians to independently double check patient identification and PCA dose settings prior to use - and each pump refill - to detect possible errors.
- Educate patients and their families about the proper use of PCA pumps. Start during the pre-operative testing visit, not after the surgery when a patient is groggy.
- Educate staff about proper use of PCA pumps. Encourage clinicians to critically think about the cumulative dose that the patient could receive if the maximum dose limits were given.

TEARING DOWN WALLS

Dan felt extremely betrayed by the healthcare industry when dealing with Diane's disabling event. Although Dan had worked in the industry as a healthcare executive recruiter, he was treated no differently than an outsider. Little was explained or discussed with him with regard to what happened to Diane.

In the end, Dan Ford has turned something tragic into something that benefits others. He has become a leader in patient safety improvement. Dan continues to speak often on the need to transform the healthcare system, and the need to embrace patients and families when medical errors occur. As a result of his experiences and work, Dan has summarized the needed changes in a list of basic principals.

1. Patient safety is a human rights issue.
2. Senior leadership has to set the standard, model, lead and guide patient safety.
3. Trust between patient and provider is fundamental; there must be underlying trust.
4. Empower the patient.
5. Encourage and support patient advocates, whether they are family, friends or others.
6. Implement hospital patient and family advisory councils. Invite patients and family members to serve on committees, including patient safety and quality committees.
7. When things go wrong, including a sentinel event, immediately take responsibility, apologize, be candid, transparent and honest about what happened. Be open to questions and repeated questions, be they big or small. This involvement and participation will be a worthy investment for all concerned. These are the right things to do.
8. Involve patients and families in the error investigations or the root cause analysis.
9. Be attentive and responsive to patient and family complaints.
10. Empower teamwork. Critical linkage of cultural leadership and teamwork is essential (aviation and the space industry are good role models).
11. Be receptive to patients' questions to care providers, such as "Did you wash your hands?" Questions like this should be taken seriously, and addressed. This helps to break down communication barriers between patients and healthcare professionals.
12. Increase the use of Rapid Response Teams.

Use of PCA pumps:
- Ask for written instructions on the use of your PCA pump.
- When using a PCA pump, you should feel steady pain relief of 0-3 on a scale of 1-10.
- If you feel extremely groggy or have trouble waking up, notify your nurse immediately. Inform your family to do the same.
- Ask your nurse to periodically check to make sure your pump is performing properly.
- Learn what pain medication is being administered and how much. Make sure your pump is performing properly.
- Ask if the unit you are on stocks Narcan, and does the staff know where it is located.
- Never let anyone else push your medication release button for you.

Food and Drug Administration (FDA) PCA Pump Recalls:
- Date: April 26, 2006
  - Product: Baxter AP II Pain Management System
  - Contact Details: http://www.accessdata.fda.gov/scripts/cdrh/cfdocs/cfRes/res.cfm?ID=43326
- Date: January 28, 2006
  - Product: Baxter 6060 Multi-Therapy Infusion Pump - Product Codes 2M9832, 2M9832P and 2M9832R; and Sabratek 6060 Homerun Infusion Pumps - Product Codes 606000, 606000-40, 606000-40L, and 606000-40I; Manufactured by an affiliate of Baxter Healthcare Corp., Deerfield, IL 60013 USA, in Singapore
  - Contact Details: http://www.accessdata.fda.gov/scripts/cdrh/cfdocs/cfRes/res.cfm?ID=42919
- Date Posted: August 16, 2005
  - Product: Syndeo PCA Syringe Pump - Product Codes

2L3113 and 2L3113R; Baxter Healthcare Corporation, Medication Delivery Division, Deerfield, IL 60015 U.S.A., pumps made in Singapore.
   ° Contact Details: http://www.accessdata.fda.gov/scripts/cdrh/ cfdocs/cfRes/res.cfm?ID=40398
• MedWatch Reports to the Food and Drug Administration (FDA)
   ° To report problems with an infusion pump contact MedWatch FDA at 1-800-FDA-1088
• For more information on PCA Pumps
   ° http://www.ismp.org/newsletters/acutecare/articles/ 20030724.asp

CHAPTER 5

THE PROMISE

In this chapter
- Find out what specialists your hospital's emergency department (ED) must have available on-call.
- What back-up plans hospitals must implement if an on-call specialist can't be reached in an emergency.
- Learn what EMTALA laws are, what they cover and how they protect your access to emergency care.

Why the absence of specialized care in the Emergency Room (ER) can matter to you?
When a hospital offers care in a particular medical specialty, such as neurosurgery or orthopedic surgery, they must have specialists in that field on-call for emergencies at all times. When a critically ill patient requiring a specialist arrives in the emergency department and the physician on-call can't be reached, hospitals must have back-up plans in place. Without such provisions, precious time is lost and the results can be devastating.

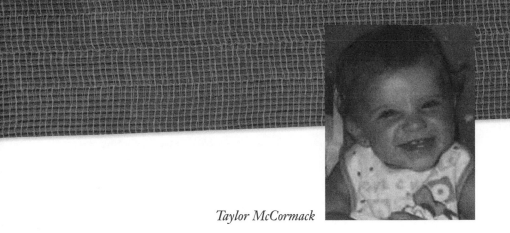

Taylor McCormack

John McCormack held the 9 mm Smith and Wesson revolver in his right hand, as he sat in front of the grave at the cemetery. There were no other people around. It would be quick and easy, easier than living with the constant anguish and grief. What a relief it would be to be free. A cold breeze came up, but John didn't move to pull his jacket tighter around him. In fact, he didn't even notice the chill. He reached out to touch the gravestone with his free hand, so large and rough, and with work-worn fingers he traced the letters and numbers that were etched on it. *Taylor Catherine McCormack*, it read, *August 23, 1999 – October 6, 2000.*

"I'm sorry," he whispered through his tears, his nose running from the crying and the cold. "I'm sorry I let you down. Daddy loves you, baby." He brushed his nose and upper lip on the sleeve of his jacket. The wind chapped his wet face. He came here often in the months since Taylor's death, but today he brought his pistol. John had spent his adult life being strong, serving and protecting people, first in the military during Desert Storm and later as a cop. He believed he was supposed to protect Taylor; it was his duty as her father. Now he considered himself a failure because he hadn't been able to prevent her death.

John was a broad-shouldered man with an easy-going manner and a thick Boston accent, who believed in treating people as he would want to be treated. As a Massachusetts state trooper, John had seen his share of misery. There were the car accidents and injuries, some of them so bad that the victims didn't make it. He had seen neglected children, and wives who had been abused by their husbands. A few times he had been the one to notify people about the death of their loved one from drugs or accidents, and had to steel himself against the look of abject horror and agony in their faces.

Cops often saw things no one should have to see. That was the dark part of the job, and John knew it before going into police work. It was a burden they carried for the public. They developed a protective shield of professional detachment that allowed them to do what they had to do, and still carry on. But it was different when it was your own child. There was no shield, no barrier, to insulate you from the pain.

John was so proud when his wife, Catherine, gave birth to Taylor. They already had two active, rambunctious boys. He would enjoy having a little girl to spoil and dote on. Taylor was a beautiful baby, despite the health issue that was discovered shortly after she was born. When Taylor was only two days old, doctors said they had a concern. Her head was larger than it should be, and they strongly suspected she had congenital hydrocephalus, a buildup of fluid in the brain ventricles, which is caused by abnormal development in the womb. It often goes hand-in-hand with other birth defects like spina bifida, but not in Taylor's case. The excess fluid begins to push the brain outward and makes the head appear large. If the condition isn't quickly diagnosed and treated, it can lead to brain damage.

Taylor was transferred to Children's Hospital, where they were better equipped to help newborns with serious health problems. Doctors used a CT scan and an MRI to measure the size of the ventricles in Taylor's brain, and the tests confirmed their suspicions of hydrocephalus. The good news, doctors told John and Catherine, was that they had caught this early and it was treatable. Also, Taylor had none of the other disabilities associated with the condition, and she was healthy in every other way. If they inserted a shunt to drain the fluid and reduce the pressure, Taylor would likely be just fine and lead a normal life.

At five days old Taylor underwent surgery to insert a shunt, a flexible tube, leading from her brain to her belly. This would allow the excess fluid to drain off from the brain into the abdomen, where it would be reabsorbed by the body. No one would even be able to tell from looking at her that the device was implanted. The operation went smoothly, and the doctors taught John and Catherine the signs and symptoms to watch out for in the event that the shunt might not be working properly. They were instructed that if they noticed increased irritability, prolonged crying, a fever or an increase in the size of Taylor's head, it was an indication that there could be trouble with the implanted shunt.

During the next year, Taylor was a constant source of entertainment for her older brother Jack, who was seven, as well as four-year-old Steven. They affectionately called her "Tay Tay." Like any younger sibling, she worked at keeping up with the big kids, attempting to do things as early as possible so she wouldn't be left out. By 13 months, she was trying to sing along with pop songs on the radio, and she pretended to read her baby books like she saw her brothers do with their stories. She learned to scoot as a form of locomotion so she could get to where she wanted to be, close to the action. She was a strawberry blonde confection, charming everyone with her ready smile and limitless energy. That first year there was only one occasion when Taylor had a medical problem. When she was eight months old, she developed a slight blockage in her shunt. A doctor made some adjustments to the shunt, and afterward she was fine.

John vividly remembers the day this tragic journey began. It was Saturday, September 30, 2000, and the whole family was in the middle of a busy weekend like so many other growing families. Jack had a hockey game, and since John's shift didn't begin until 3:00 that afternoon the games were a family affair for John and Catherine. Steven enjoyed the games, but Taylor was little. She didn't have the patience and there wasn't much for a toddler to do. It was better to leave her with Grandma, Catherine's mother, where she could play and take a nap. Catherine and John dropped her and left with the boys for the afternoon. Catherine had noticed that the day before that Taylor had seemed tired, but it could be something as simple as teething or coming down with the sniffles.

As the day passed, Taylor became more lethargic. When Grandma gave her some juice to drink she vomited, and was unable to keep any food or liquid down. Catherine arrived to pick up Taylor shortly before dinner time, and was instantly concerned. Catherine called their pediatrician, who advised her to call the hospital. A Dr. Cho at the Children's Hospital told Catherine to wait until Monday, it was probably nothing. But clearly something wasn't right. Following her own instincts, Catherine left the boys with her mother around 6:30 that evening and headed out for the emergency room at the local Children's Hospital.

As the staff examined Taylor in the ER, they asked Catherine questions about her baby's symptoms and behavior over the last 24 hours. They ordered tests on blood gas levels, and Taylor squirmed a little, but didn't cry as they took blood samples. Even when they put in an IV, she was docile and quiet. Catherine helped to comfort Taylor by stroking her head and softly singing to her.

A neurosurgery resident was paged, and several minutes later a doctor entered the exam area, introducing himself as Dr. Cho, the doctor Catherine had spoken with earlier. After a brief examination, he told Catherine that Taylor's shunt was blocked; he would have to tap the shunt. He asked for a sterile tray, and told Catherine she would have to leave while they did the procedure. Catherine called John at work, and by 10:30 he was there with her. They waited together, hoping to hear that everything had been corrected and Taylor would be fine.

The minutes stacked up as John and Catherine became more anxious. A nurse in scrubs emerged from the treatment area and approached them in the waiting room. She asked them to come back and talk with the doctor. As the McCormack's entered Taylor's room, they could see the serious look on Dr. Cho's face. He broke the unexpected news that Taylor's shunt was failing. When he tapped the shunt it was dry, and her condition was deteriorating.

"Your daughter will need to go to surgery tonight. I've called the neurosurgeon and contacted the OR," he said, before giving them a moment to digest the information.

"Is she going to be okay?" John asked.

"If we do the surgery tonight, she'll be home by Monday," Dr. Cho assured them.

For the next couple of hours John and Catherine took turns cradling Taylor, waiting for the neurosurgeon to show up and end their daughter's discomfort. Taylor whimpered occasionally, raising her hand to her head and rubbing it, or gently pulling at the sticky bandage covering her IV. As time went on, she became quiet and glassy-eyed. *What if the surgeon doesn't get here soon,* John wondered to himself, but he didn't say it out loud for fear of upsetting Catherine even more. They both had unspoken fears they were keeping to themselves, afraid that if they gave those thoughts a voice it would make things worse. Finally Taylor drifted off into a fitful sleep, exhausted by the pain and all the poking and prodding.

For the umpteenth time, John asked the nurse what was taking so long. When would the neurosurgeon get there? Although she was calmer than John, the nurse seemed just as frustrated as he did. John heard her outside the doorway, quietly telling someone they had paged the surgeon several times and he hadn't answered. There was no back-up pediatric neurosurgeon on call. Just after midnight, Dr. Cho told them he had a room for Taylor on the medical unit, and they could take her there now.

"Why isn't she going to surgery? You said she needed surgery tonight," John demanded, his voice rising louder with frustration.

"There's no OR available," Dr. Cho replied." There were other surgeries on the schedule that were more urgent. We'll admit her for the night and take her to surgery by 8:00 tomorrow morning. She'll be fine," the resident tried to sound sure. The nurse shook her head disapprovingly.

John was uncomfortable with this change in plans, but figured they knew what they were doing. He had always trusted doctors. *They'll take such good care of Taylor,* he thought. After all, this was one of the finest children's hospitals in the country, right? At 12:20 they moved Taylor up to a room on the fifth floor for the night. John stayed at the hospital through most of the night with Catherine and Taylor.

Catherine curled up in the big chair next to Taylor's crib and allowed herself to doze off and on. Her head jerked up as she awoke at 2:00 that morning, when Taylor yelled out, "Mama," before falling back asleep. She stood next to the crib for awhile and watched Taylor breathe and dream before going back to the chair. In the wee hours of the morning John left for Catherine's mother's house, to check on the boys.

It was hard to tell how much time had passed when she came to again. Catherine's eyes struggled to adjust as she looked at the clock on the wall. It was just after 6:00 in the morning. The sun would be coming up in another half-hour, and they would be getting Taylor ready for surgery soon. Catherine rose and went to the crib. She gently touched her baby, but got no response. Something was wrong. She looked at Taylor and flipped on the lights. Taylor was blue. Catherine ran out into the hall and began yelling for someone to come, "She's blue! Someone help me, my baby's blue!"

A nurse and a doctor, both in scrubs, ran into the room and looked at Taylor. The doctor grabbed her shoulders and shook her. "Call a code," he told the nurse.

"Push the code button. It's by you," the nurse said.

"Where is it? I can't find it."

Catherine looked on in disbelief. Her baby needed emergency help, and they were fumbling around trying to find buttons. The nurse pointed to a button on the wall over by the doctor. He awkwardly reached out and pressed it. Minutes later the crash cart and code team finally arrived, and at last the doctor began CPR.

John received a call from Catherine at 6:20 that morning regarding the code and returned in a hurry. As he entered Taylor's room on the fifth floor, the staff was still working on Taylor, trying to give her oxygen. He watched them squeezing a bag in and out to force air into her little lungs, and whispered, "Daddy's here. Keep on fighting. I'm here now." The doctor was there quizzing Catherine about what time all of this had happened.

Taylor had a tube in her throat and was hooked up to monitors. They tried to get John to go out to the nurses' station, but it was difficult to make him budge. He was pleading with them to do something more for his little girl. A lady was there attempting to comfort his wife, who was nearly hysterical. She spoke in a soothing voice and had her arm around Catherine's shoulder.

The staff escorted the family into a small waiting room. Dr. Nathan, another pediatric neurologist, was called in to perform surgery on Taylor. Just 45 minutes later, Dr. Nathan and Dr. Cho came out to speak to John and Catherine. The doctors told them that there was a buildup of carbon dioxide in Taylor's bloodstream, and that had caused her to stop breathing.

"So what the hell does that mean? Is Taylor going to make it?" John asked hopefully.

Dr. Cho wouldn't make eye contact with them, and looked down at the floor as if he was carefully studying something on the carpet. The color had drained from his face and he looked pale. They were running tests on her brain activity, including an emergency CAT scan, Dr. Nathan told them, but it didn't look good. She had been without oxygen too long, and the prognosis was poor. Taylor was in a coma, and they didn't know if she would recover.

Deep down, John knew what they were saying. You didn't need a medical degree to understand. The doctors were trying to tell them that Taylor wasn't going to get better, that she would likely not wake up. John felt the anger rising up inside of him until he thought he might explode. How could they let this happen? They could have done something and they let it happen anyway.

He left the room, afraid of the intensity of his own emotions. John stormed down the hallway toward the doors leading from the unit to the elevators, his feet hitting the floor hard and fast. Reaching the doors, he forcefully shoved them open with one quick smack, and blew up at last. All his pent up emotions erupted like a volcano. He knew people heard him, but he didn't care. Let them hear.

After taking some time to cool off, John returned to the unit. Late in the evening he asked to use the phone at the nurses' station. He needed to call Catherine's mother and their parish priest. They refused to let him use the phone there and made him go down to the pay phone in the waiting area. With no change in his pockets, John made a collect call. The staff seemed intimidated by him after his outburst. He sensed that they viewed him as a man with a temper, who had a job with a gun.

For the next several days they lived in a state of limbo, waiting for further tests. John made it clear they didn't want Dr. Cho treating their daughter any longer. During some of the tests Taylor's eyes flickered, but the doctors told John those were seizures and not a sign of improvement or brain activity. Taylor was on life support, and in an area where there was no such thing as privacy. It was next to impossible to sit with her and have a quiet, intimate moment between parents and baby.

John had heard about a healing priest in the Mission Hill area, down the street from the hospital, and he was seeking a miracle. He had Fr. McDonough come to bless and anoint Taylor as the family looked on and prayed for her recovery.

The McCormack's met with a group of doctors, who gave them the grim results from tests they performed earlier in the week. Taylor had 98 percent brain damage and was, by medical definition, brain dead. Her current condition would never change or improve, and there was no reason to hope that something might change. John wanted to believe she would still fight.

John and Catherine were torn over what they should do next. Should they keep her on life support any longer? How much longer? Although the doctors told them there was no hope, there was a part of him that just couldn't give up. They would have some agonizing decisions to make in the coming days.

John's sister, a nurse, told him to get Taylor's hospital records, and he demanded them despite arguments from doctors, staff and administrators. No matter how this ended, they wanted to get to the bottom of how this could occur in the first place. Not only did they need to know what really happened, he didn't want anyone else to suffer as they had.

He had so many questions, ones that weren't immediately answered in Taylor's records. Why didn't the neurosurgeon answer his page? Why did they say there was no operating room available later in the evening, when they originally said she needed surgery that night? Why did Dr. Cho emphasize how important quick treatment was when they first came to the ER, and then say Taylor's operation could wait until morning?

On Thursday night, John was at a Bruin's hockey game with Jack. He certainly wasn't in the mood for sports, but Jack's team had the honor of playing in the arena just before the Bruin's game. It was something Jack would always remember, and he wasn't going to deny him that special moment of excitement and joy. John felt like he was in a fog, and wished he could be more present for Jack. He worried about what this was doing to his sons.

After the game, Catherine and John gave the boys baths before bed. Jack and Steven were asking tough questions about whether Taylor was ever going to come home. In that moment, John knew what they had to do. He didn't want to put their boys through this any longer. Taylor was gone, and her body was being kept alive artificially by machines. Nothing could bring her back. To keep her like this only served to extend the misery indefinitely. Although he hated to let her go, he knew it was wrong to keep her this way.

John talked with Catherine after the boys were in bed and they came to the same conclusion; it was best to take her off life-support. It was the right thing to do. They called the doctor and hospital to tell them they had made a decision, then planned for the boys to come with them and say goodbye to their sister.

It was Friday, October 6, and they all gathered in the hospital room. The chaplain from the police precinct was there, and gave Taylor a final anointing and prayers. The doctor turned off the machines that were doing the work of her organs, and aided by a nurse, unhooked the tubes and monitors so the McCormack's could hold their baby. Jack and Steven gently touched her head and her hands, and said goodbye to "Tay Tay." Steven went to the waiting area and cried quietly, but Jack lingered a little longer. He cried and whispered, "We'll always love you." She continued to take sporadic breaths for another three-and-a-half hours, as they took turns holding her in their arms. Then it was over.

They took one last set of footprints as a keepsake, a precious memento, and then John asked Catherine to take the boys and leave. He didn't want them to be there when the staff from the morgue arrived, but he felt compelled to stay there and make sure everything was done right, with care and dignity.

A worker from the morgue brought up a little tray on a cart, the right size for a small child, and a white cloth to wrap her in. John said he wanted to carry his daughter down to the morgue instead. He asked to help, and began to wrap Taylor in the white cloth. There was laughter on the other side of the closed door, nurses sharing a joke, and it felt like a personal insult. Leaning down, he kissed Taylor's cheek and told her he was sorry, before he finished carefully wrapping her.

Lifting her into his arms, he followed the staff member down to the morgue. John placed Taylor's body on a tray. It was freezing cold and dark. He helped the staff put the tray into the refrigerated compartment and shut the door.

Before leaving her there, he asked about arrangements. The staff said they would call the funeral director for him. He made sure to tell them that he and his wife wanted to donate some of Taylor's organs to help other children.

John spent Saturday walking the cemetery grounds looking for a funeral plot for his daughter. What could possibly be an appropriate plot for a 13-month-old girl? There was no such thing. To add to the burden, the hospital never called the funeral director, so John took care of that as well.

The funeral Mass was crowded with family and friends, but no physicians from the hospital came or sent their condolences. A few of the nurses who had cared for Taylor in the hospital came to the funeral to pay their respects. So did the obstetrician who delivered Taylor the year before. That served to let John know that there were still healthcare professionals who cared, despite the mistrust and resentment he now felt for physicians in general.

Shortly after the funeral, the hospital called and wanted to meet. John told them no. They hadn't offered any help up to this point, no support, no apologies, no regrets, just a press release. He wasn't about to make nice with them now and ease their consciences. John and Catherine had already discovered that the neurosurgeon who was on call the night they brought in Taylor claimed to have placed his pager on vibrate while he was out, then never switched the sound back on and fell asleep.

In the days after the funeral, John made more disturbing discoveries about the circumstances surrounding Taylor's care, details that had been kept quiet. Another pediatric neurosurgeon, who would have been a backup, was home with his sick child and not immediately available, but could have been called in for an emergency. The resident chose not to contact that physician, because he didn't want to risk getting in trouble with a superior for disturbing him. Dr. Cho's medical license had expired at midnight, and he was no longer legally able to practice medicine at that point. John and Catherine were told that no operating rooms were available, when actually there were two separate OR units that could have been used.

John felt completely betrayed by the people and the facility that they believed would help them. The hospital had gambled with his daughter's life, and then lied about it to protect their interests. The McCormack's filed formal complaints with the Massachusetts Department of Public Health (DPH), and the Board of Registration in Medicine. The investigation would take many months to reach a conclusion.

In the meantime, nothing could ease the pain and anger at those who harmed Taylor, or the anger and guilt he felt towards himself. Their baby was helpless and trusted him completely. Privately, he blamed himself for not protecting his daughter. That was a father's job in his eyes, to protect his children, and by his own measure he had failed. In the months right after Taylor's death those feelings gnawed at him, eating holes in his soul, until the pain was too much to live with any longer.

On his first day back to preschool after Taylor's death, four-year-old Steven told John he had a great idea. He asked his daddy to get out the ladder, so he could climb up to heaven and put a Band-aid on Taylor's head. Then she would be fixed and could come back home. The words to describe John's pain didn't even exist. He didn't know how much more he could take.

John sat by Taylor's grave and poured his heart out, apologizing yet again for his imagined sins. The gun rested in his lap. When he said everything he had come there to say, he raised the pistol to his head and positioned it against his temple. He took a long deep breath, what he thought would be his last one.

A cold breeze came up again, and suddenly John felt a gentle nudge on his back. Somehow, he knew he wasn't alone; Taylor was there. He felt it. Her presence surrounded him. Uninvited thoughts came into his head, images of Catherine and the boys. It was Taylor's way of communicating with him, he felt sure. And he knew he couldn't do this. This wasn't the legacy he wanted to leave his boys. They needed him. He was their father, too, not just Taylor's, and he didn't have the right to take that away from them. Jack and Steven deserved to have a father. John lowered the gun.

As he sat there trying to make sense of what had just happened, John made a solemn promise to Taylor. He vowed he would do everything in his power to make sure this didn't happen to other kids. From here on he would work to change things, to make hospitals safer for children. He wasn't sure what that would entail, but whatever it took, it was a challenge he was accepting. It would give some meaning to an otherwise meaningless tragedy.

July, 2004, Boston, Massachusetts

A big, burly man wearing a sandwich board moved through the crowd outside the convention center in Boston. It was the 2004 Democratic convention, where delegates would go through the formality of choosing a presidential candidate. When he spoke, the man had an accent that let people know he was a native. His broad smile and firm handshake quickly put others at ease, although a closer look revealed deep sadness in his eyes.

The man, John McCormack, passed out brochures and books on patient safety, and he told anyone who would listen about his daughter, Taylor, and the medical errors that took her life. He was eager to talk about the bill he was trying to get passed through the Massachusetts state legislature. The bill was called Taylor's Law, and would mandate that victims of medical errors have the right to give testimony to the review boards that conduct hearings and make decisions about disciplinary action. These victim impact statements would give patients and their families a voice in the proceedings.

John's sandwich board displayed pictures of Taylor in a pumpkin suit, at the beach and with her doll, as well as mind-boggling statistics about deadly medical errors. He was fearless, approaching news anchors and political pundits from the major networks, senators and congressmen from Capitol Hill and consumer advocates from around the country. He could be seen on the outdoor news sets the networks set up, or in Faneuil Hall where everyone went to eat and shop. Taylor gave him the strength to do it.

Then he went to New York in August for the Republican convention, and did it all over again. This was a bipartisan issue. Medical errors make no distinction for political party.

He began campaigning for patient safety reform in 2002, just as he promised Taylor he would. Connecting with other patient safety advocates and groups, John's story was quickly picked up by the press and national political figures took notice. In July, 2003, he went to Capitol Hill carrying a portable TV with a videotape of Taylor in it, and he spoke to Congress about his family's experience, bringing many to tears. In 2004, John watched as Governor Mitt Romney signed Taylor's Law after it was passed unanimously in the legislature.

John is still working for patients' safety and rights, but that's not the only addition to his legacy since that day in the cemetery. Four years after Taylor's death, Catherine gave birth to Colleen Marie McCormack on October 8, 2004, a beautiful and healthy baby girl.

KEEPING HIS PROMISE

John McCormack has kept his promise to Taylor many times over. After her death, he embarked on a mission. At the time, John had no connection with people in the patient safety movement, but that didn't stop him. As a law enforcement officer he knew his rights, and he made it his business to draw critical attention to the crisis of medical errors. He not only appeared at the political conventions in 2004, but at the Massachusetts Board of Registration.

John continues to fight tirelessly, and most recently has worked with the Massachusetts Nursing Association to improve the nurse-to-patient ratios in hospitals. Many states have enacted a one-nurse-to-five-patient ratio to improve patient safety. Some states without a ratio law have hospitals that voluntarily limit ratios, but without a state law, hospitals can have dangerously high levels of patients for each nurse.

Even now, for the McCormack family, talking about broken systems doesn't take away the pain of losing their little girl. But it does help to understand that hospitals need healing, and the fragmented systems will continue to harm people until those systems are repaired.

Throughout that first night in the hospital, the neurosurgery resident and emergency room staff repeatedly paged the on-call neurosurgeon. The multiple pages went unanswered, as the McCormack's later learned, because he had switched it to vibrate and fell asleep. He never responded to the life-threatening emergency.

Taylor's medical emergency is not an uncommon one for children with neuron-shunts. Any hospital in the U.S. that provides neurosurgical services can deal with a blocked shunt. The Children's Hospital failed to provide the basic treatment and life support that Taylor needed, simply because all their systems depended on one person. That person failed them, and no backup systems were in place to rescue Taylor.

Although the resident attempted to "tap" and unblock the shunt, he was not qualified or experienced enough to perform the immediate surgery that would repair or replace Taylor's shunt and save her life.

In addition, even though John and Catherine were told an operating room was not available, it was later discovered that this was not true. When the McCormack's brought legal action against the hospital, an operating room nurse who had been on duty the night Taylor came in testified in a deposition that an operating room was available. If the on-call neurosurgeon had come to the hospital, he could have performed surgery to relieve the swelling in Taylor's brain.

There were other failures. Although the resident and staff continued to page the neurosurgeon, apparently they

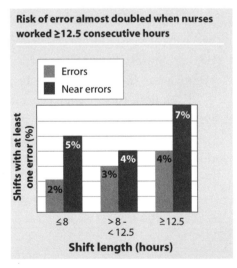

Risk of error almost doubled when nurses worked ≥12.5 consecutive hours

Source: Scott LD, Rogers AE, Hwang WT, Zhang Y. Effects of critical care nurses' work hours on vigilance and patients' safety. Am J Crit Care. 2006; 15: 30-37.

never called his home or cell phone numbers. The multiple lab tests they performed on Taylor were not evaluated in a timely fashion, and while the correct tests were done, the doctors and nurses did not provide treatment based on the test results. Blood gasses drawn on Taylor indicated she had elevated carbon dioxide levels in her bloodstream, but no one responded to the results in time to save her life.

One of the biggest mistakes was neglecting to place Taylor in pediatric intensive care unit, where she would have had minute by minute monitoring of her breathing and other vital signs. They should have recognized that she was far too sick to be on a regular medical floor. And even on the medical floor where she was placed, heart and breathing monitors could have been used to alert nurses that she was in trouble.

Regardless of where the blame is placed, the bottom line is that people and systems failed, leading to Taylor's tragic, needless death. There was a cascade of events without a safety net. Each process failed with no backup to stop these breakdowns. All the while, her parents, who had been taught to trust the healthcare systems, were victims of these very systems that were designed to heal.

Taylor's death places a spotlight on the fragmented and broken systems present in our hospitals. The Massachusetts Department of Public Health substantiated the multiple problems that contributed to Taylor's death, confirming that she should have been in an ICU, and that the hospital failed to respond to critical tests.

The McCormack case caused the hospital to reevaluate their practices and make policy changes. According to John McCormack, Dr. Nathan, who was called in to operate on Taylor after her respiratory arrest, told John and Catherine, "Our hospital failed you, and they have to change their policies and procedures."

Although the hospital was shocked and traumatized over Taylor's death, they had subsequent events later on. The death of a 5-year-old boy with epilepsy triggered a federal review of the hospital's eligibility for Medicare and Medicaid funding, after investigators found that numerous doctors and nurses failed to intervene and stop the boy's severe seizures. According to a report, medical personnel failed to call their supervisors to raise questions and save his life.

CONFIDENTIAL JUSTICE FOR THE DOCTORS

The neurosurgeon on call, the resident physician on duty and a senior resident who had been advising the resident by phone, all faced disciplinary action by the Massachusetts Medical Board, known as the Board of Registration.

Physicians' disciplinary hearings are private, and protected by law from the public, treated much like personnel issues instead of matters of public safety. When the McCormack's wanted to attend, they were barred from the hearings, and only allowed to write a letter to the board. Each doctor received a letter of warning that went into their files at the Medical Board. All of the doctors continue to practice medicine today.

Being barred from these hearings only added insult to injury, and started John McCormack on a path to enact a new law in honor of Taylor. John fought for four years, campaigning to pass this measure. In conjunction with his state senator, Therese Murray, they worked to construct a law that gives families like the McCormack's new rights of participation at Medical Board hearings. The bill, called Taylor's Law, allows patients and their families to make a victim impact statement and to bring an attorney to the hearings. Passed in Massachusetts in 2004, John would now like to see this provision become law at the federal level, or at least passed by other states.

PROTECT YOURSELF IN TODAY'S HEALTHCARE SYSTEM

Many emergency departments provide excellent care, however it's important to be aware of possible dangers when entering an emergency department (ED). Because these units deal with sicker patients than traditional medical units, they must often perform larger volumes of tests, exchange more extensive amounts

$5.6 Million

THE DOLLAR NUMBER IN FINES IMPOSED ON U.S. HOSPITALS FOR VIOLATING EMTALA LAW BETWEEN 1995-2000

(*Source: U.S. General Accounting Office, Report to Congressional Committees, Emergency Care, EMTALA, June 2001.*)

of information between healthcare professionals, perform more procedures and administer more medication. With this high level of activity and intensive services, the chance for medical errors increases dramatically.

The Emergency Medical Treatment and Active Labor Act (EMTALA) is a law that oversees how a patient with an unstable condition may be treated, refused treatment or transferred from one hospital to another. EMTALA was passed in 1986 as part of Medicare legislation. Although the law originally applied to Medicare patients, the statute has become the gold standard for how hospitals treat patients. All hospitals that receive Medicare patients must comply with this law, which includes most hospitals in the U.S. While the main purpose of the law was to keep hospitals from "dumping" patients, there is a key component of the law that sets standards for unstable patients in emergency departments.

The law states that any patient who comes to the emergency department requesting an examination or treatment for a medical condition must be provided with an appropriate medical screening exam, to determine if he or she is suffering from an "emergency medical condition." If the patient is found to have such a condition, then the hospital is obligated to either provide them with treatment until they are stable, or transfer the patient to another hospital, in conformance with the statute's directives.

Taylor was clearly suffering from an unstable medical condition, but since they treated her, how did the hospital violate the statute? The law also imposes a firm duty to institute treatment if an emergency medical condition does exist. The children's hospital had neurosurgery as a listed service, so the hospital was obligated to provide a safe and reliable execution of these services. In Taylor's case, the hospital violated EMTALA by not having an available neurosurgeon.

It is critical to understand that a hospital must provide the services it lists under its license. A patient in unstable condition who is turned away or delayed treatment because a specialty physician is not available is in direct violation of EMTALA. There are immediate and costly fines associated with EMTALA violations, starting at $50,000. A hospital may also risk losing its Medicare funding if it is in direct violation, which in most cases will result in closing down a hospital. Additionally, there is a section in the law that imposes a penalty on a physician who fails to respond to an emergency situation when he is assigned as the on-call physician. The children's hospital was under an EMTALA evaluation stemming from the case of the boy who died from seizures.

HOW YOU CAN APPLY THE PROTECTION

It is important to understand EMTALA and your rights related to this federal law. In the event that you or a family member has an unstable condition, and the hospital provides a specialty service related to that medical condition, then the hospital is obligated to have the on-call physician or a physician of the same specialty come to the hospital and treat the patient.

You can insist that the specialty physician treat you or your family member, and if there is a delay, you can demand another physician of the same specialty, or insist on a safe transfer to a hospital that provides the same services.

If you are having a delay in services, just mentioning that you understand EMTALA, pronounced "em-tal-ah," may move the hospital into immediate action. You can also insist the hospital administrator, chief medical officer or the chief of staff be contacted immediately to resolve the situation.

When in the Emergency Department (ED):
- Ask the emergency department physician to review all tests with you. Test results are processed quickly in the emergency department, usually within one to three hours maximum.
- Ask what each test result means and what follow-up is necessary.
- If you are having difficulty obtaining needed emergency treatment at a hospital, make sure the emergency department staff know you understand your rights under EMTALA, the Emergency Medical Treatment and Active Labor Act.
- EMTALA mandates that licensed emergency departments must have on-call specialty physicians and surgeons available 24 hours a day, seven days a week for all of its licensed services, or provide safe, appropriate transfer to another facility in critical situations if they do not provide the service a patient must have.
- Contact your physician to involve them in treatment decisions, if possible. They can provide valuable input about your medical history or condition, and may act as an advocate with emergency physicians on your behalf.
- If you have serious concerns that are not being addressed, ask to speak to the Chief of Emergency Medicine at the hospital.

Resources for you:
- To report an EMTALA violation, go to:
  - http://www.medlaw.com/healthlaw/EMTALA/reporting/index.shtml
- For more information on Taylor's Law, visit:
  - http://memorial2taylor.com/
- For more information on nursing ratios in Massachusetts, visit:
  - http://www.massnurses.org/news/2006/04/taylors_law2.htm

CHAPTER 6

COMING

In this chapter
- Find out what medically-induced trauma (MIT) is, and how it can affect both you and care providers involved.
- Discover what help is available to treat medically-induced trauma.
- Learn how to help decrease your risk for anesthesia-related complications during surgery.

Why the effects of medically induced trauma are important for you to know about?

When a patient suffers an unintended adverse event or experiences an unplanned medical event, the physical and psychological impact can run deep and affect the well-being of the victim and their family members. To complicate matters, the patient must continue to seek treatment and care from the very system that harmed them. The process of coping and learning to trust again can be difficult.

TOGETHER

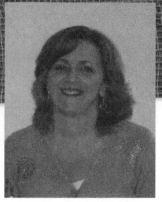

Linda Kenney

It was a Thursday morning, and Linda Kenney was getting set to have yet another orthopedic procedure that day.

"There's no sense in you waiting around here. You might as well take off and come back later," she reassured her husband, Kevin, as a nurse finished prepping her for surgery.

After 19 surgeries this scene had become familiar for Linda and Kevin Kenney. Her multiple surgeries were just another part of their lives, and this surgery for an ankle replacement would be number 20. Born with bilateral club feet, Linda had undergone one operation after another to correct the condition. They had become accustomed to the process of surgery and recovery. There was no reason to think this procedure would be unusual in any way for the 37-year-old wife and mother. If she was going to be unconscious for the next few hours, Linda didn't want Kevin to be sitting in the waiting room, bored and uncomfortable. He leaned over the gurney as she drew his face close with her hands to kiss him goodbye, and Kevin said he would see her when she woke up.

Once Kevin was out of sight Linda looked up at Dr. Walker, the anesthesiologist, who had just arrived. "I'm a little nervous," she confessed to him. Although she'd been through these things before, this was the first time they were using an anesthetic nerve block along with the general anesthesia. They had discussed it in his office, but for some reason she felt apprehensive.

Several gurneys with patients were lined up against the wall, ready to go, in the preop holding area at the busy Boston hospital. It would be Linda's turn next. Dr. Walker began to administer the nerve block so she would be set to enter the operating room. That was the last thing she would remember from that day.

A moment later, Linda became disoriented, and then began having a grand mal seizure. Her eyes rolled back in her head and her body jerked uncontrollably on the gurney. Then everything stopped. She was in full cardiac arrest. The doctor called a code and an emergency team came immediately, but Linda wasn't responding to the electrical shocks or injections of drugs to start her heart. Other patients waiting for surgery were looking on, horrified by what they were seeing.

Somehow the nerve block had accidentally gone into Linda's blood stream instead of the nerves in her ankle, stopping her heart. Despite Dr. Walker's vast experience and attention to detail, something went wrong. They had to get the Bupivacaine, the anesthetic drug he used, out of her system or she would die.

By an amazing stroke of luck or blessing, an open-heart surgical suite was across the hall, empty. It had been prepared for a scheduled cardiac bypass surgery that morning, but the patient wasn't there yet. The sophisticated cardiopulmonary bypass equipment was primed and set to go. A decision was quickly made, and the team working on Linda wheeled her in there for emergency bypass to keep her alive. They had just minutes to get her on the heart-lung machine before it would be too late.

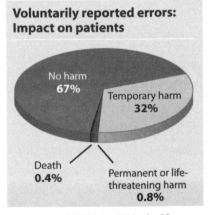

Voluntarily reported errors: Impact on patients

No harm 67%
Temporary harm 32%
Death 0.4%
Permanent or life-threatening harm 0.8%

Source: Milch CE, Salem DN, Pauker SG, Lundquist TG, Kumar S, Chen J. Voluntary electronic reporting of medical errors and adverse events. J Gen Intern Med. 2005 Dec 22

In an act that was violent but crucial, the scalpel cut sharply and precisely down the front of Linda's chest, then a doctor opened the sternum and ribcage to gain access to her paralyzed heart. A pump with a centrifuge would do the work of her heart for the time being, forcing the blood through her body as it cleansed the toxic drug from her system.

A little over an hour later, they were able to start weaning Linda off the bypass machine. A specialized open-heart anesthesiologist continued to maintain her breathing tube and a central IV line they had placed during the crisis. When the doctors finished the procedure and let Dr Walker know that they had been successful, he breathed deeply, sighing as he became aware of the tension in his body for the first time that morning.

The hospital repeatedly tried to reach Kevin, but couldn't locate him. He had thought this was a day surgery, and planned to return when Linda was out of the recovery room and he could be with her. Only able to reach Kevin's voicemail, the orthopedic surgeon left a message. "Please call the hospital so I can give you some information about your wife."

Linda was moved immediately following the surgery to the Intensive Care Unit. Dr. Walker was determined to track Linda's progress. He felt a tremendous responsibility for what had happened. As Linda was wheeled off to the cardiac ICU, a clerk informed Dr. Walker that Kevin was in the waiting area. The orthopedic surgeon and Dr. Walker decided they would talk to him together.

The staff had placed Kevin in a tiny private waiting room for families, containing two uncomfortable chairs and a small table. He was nervously pacing in what little space there was. Both doctors peered through the window in the door and saw a short man with a sturdy, athletic build. Although he had a boyish Irish face, his salt-and-pepper hair gave away the fact that he was in his mid-forties. They could see the worry in his expression.

As the two doctors entered the room, Linda's husband asked, "Did you fix her up?" He looked at the doctors expectantly, waiting for some assurance from them.

The orthopedic surgeon began. "There were complications. We had to crack open her chest."

Kevin's reaction was swift and instinctive. He lunged at the anesthesiologist. "What did you do to my beautiful wife?" he shouted, as he tried to grab the doctor. As Kevin went for Dr. Walker, the orthopedic surgeon struggled to get between them and push Kevin away. He managed to wedge himself in, as Kevin's voice grew louder and his language more threatening. At last Kevin stopped struggling, and dissolved into tears. He settled on the edge of one of the chairs and held his head in his hands as they tried to explain to him what had happened. Although he appeared calmer now, Kevin was still fuming as he listened. If these doctors only understood, he thought; his wife was his world.

They told him about the injection of the anesthetic, describing Linda's reaction and telling Kevin it was a rare complication of the medication, a reaction of some sort. Dr. Walker focused on the technical explanation, attempting to remain clinical and detached from the situation. It was the only way he could hide his own overwhelming emotions surrounding the dramatic event. Inside, the incident had deeply shaken him, and he still felt wobbly with the knowledge of how close they had come to loosing Linda.

Kevin wondered what he would say to their three children. Their 13-year-old son and 12-year-old daughter would be able to understand some of this, but their baby girl was only three and would never grasp why Mommy wasn't there. They had just moved the family to their dream house in a suburb of Boston. Linda and Kevin barely even knew their neighbors. Despite that, he phoned one of the new neighbors and asked her to look after the kids, telling her about their situation. He was told not to worry about a thing. The kids would stay with her family for the night.

The orthopedic surgeon escorted Kevin up to the cardiac ICU to see Linda and speak with the cardiac surgeon. The surgeon was brutally honest, telling him Linda's chances for making it through the night were fifty-fifty. Kevin stayed with her through the night, calming her when she became agitated and restless. At one point, she started to crash again, and the nurse assured Kevin she was "going to land her like a 747." The fact that the nurse was firm in her conviction made Kevin feel more confident about the outcome.

On the second day, Dr. Walker attempted to see how Linda was doing. He was wracked with concern over what had happened, and apprehensive for her welfare. At Kevin's request, he was blocked from having any contact with Linda. But when Dr. Walker was informed by the staff that Linda's husband was in the hospital, and did he want to speak with him, he took a chance and went to see him. Despite Kevin's anger about what had happened to his wife, he did see the doctor briefly. He apologized to Dr. Walker for his initial reaction the day before, and outstretched his hand for him to shake.

Kevin had not forgiven the doctor, and still held him responsible for Linda's condition, but his wife's trauma was bad enough without compounding the problem by behaving badly.

Linda remained sedated and on a ventilator in the cardiac ICU for the next few days. Their family's personal support system was enormous. At one point there were 25 people in the waiting room, all there for Linda. Her mother and seven aunts came to help. Neighbors and relatives pitched in to help with the three kids and the house. But even with all the help, it wasn't the same as having Linda handling things. There were inevitable gaps, as Kevin discovered the day their three-year-old was left at preschool because no one remembered to pick her up.

Despite help and concern from the people in their lives, Kevin still felt overwhelmed emotionally by what they were all going through. It seemed to him that no one really understood. Unfortunately, the hospital offered no assistance with that aspect of their situation. No organized support was available to guide him through these unexpected and unfamiliar circumstances.

Meanwhile, Jason Walker was still reeling from the experience as well. Linda was his patient, and she had placed her trust in him. The responsibility he felt for what happened to her weighed heavily on him, and he so wanted to find out how Linda was doing and let her know he was sorry. But the system was designed to keep that from ever happening. Kevin wasn't the only person to block his access to her; the hospital was strongly discouraging any contact between Jason and his former patient. They were concerned about liability and litigation, and wanted him to remain silent and distant. The walls went up on both sides, as everyone staked out their ground. Oddly, there was no organized support for doctors who went through an adverse event like this, any more than there was for patients and families. The hospital wanted him to get back in there and do his job, and so that's what he did. A day after the incident, he was in the operating room as if nothing had ever happened.

Four days after that terrifying moment outside of the operating room, Linda was finally transferred from the cardiac ICU into a hospital room. For the first time since the incident, she was awake and aware. The surgeon and Kevin told her what had happened that day. The last thing she remembered was saying goodbye to her husband, but she only had to look at her body to know something devastating had taken place after that. There were wires and tubes, and a sensation of heaviness on her chest. She discovered a hematoma, a huge swollen bruise, on the inside of her upper thigh, where the cardiac surgeon had gone into the groin area to insert a central IV line.

At first she didn't realize how bad she looked. Instead, she saw it in other people's eyes and in their reaction to her appearance. It was only over the next day or two that she developed a true sense of how serious things had been, and of the battering her body had endured. Alone in her hospital room, she touched her fingertips to her throat and slowly moved them downward, tracing the bandage that ran the length of her chest. It occurred to her that she would carry this emblem, this reminder, with her for the rest of her life. The enormity of it all washed over her.

Realizing that she had almost died, Linda was filled with a feeling of profound gratitude that she was still alive. Her concern now was for her husband and children. Kevin was clearly a wreck. He cried every time he looked at her, thinking of how close he had come to losing her. Linda tried to lighten the mood by joking with him. "The reason why God didn't take me," she said, "was because no one else would be able to put up with you."

Linda asked to see her chart while she was still in the hospital. She was no stranger to hospital records, because she worked as a secretary in a hospital OR unit at another facility. The account of her cardiac arrest listed an allergic reaction as the cause. She knew that was false. This was no allergy; something else had happened. They were covering their rears to protect their own interests. Eventually, before she was discharged to go home, her persistent probing led to the truth, buried in the notes the surgeon had dictated. Somehow, the Bupivacaine had gone into her bloodstream during the initiation of the nerve block and resulted in cardiac toxicity from the powerful anesthetic drug. It had immobilized her heart instantly.

For the remainder of her hospital stay, Linda had enough to do just getting from one day to the next. Coping with the pain from having her chest cracked open and her heart revived, and dealing with the indignity of having strangers help her with intimate daily tasks, was about all she could handle. She focused on getting well enough to go home to her family. After nearly dying, everything else seemed minor.

No one at the hospital talked about what happened, or mentioned the incident to her. It was like an elephant in the room. So if nobody was mentioning it, Linda concluded that maybe it wasn't a big deal. Besides, at this point she didn't have the surplus energy to think about the emotional aspect of what she had gone through. For now, she had her hands full.

Ten days after what should have been a day-surgery, the hospital discharged Linda to go home. They gave her instructions on how to care for chest incision, and information about the visiting nurse that would be checking on her. But no one prepared her for the emotional fallout she and her family might experience. There were no instructions on how to move forward after an event like this. The hospital didn't send home any phone numbers or resources to contact for the emotional and psychological recovery.

In the following days, each member of the family dealt with the aftermath in a different way. Kevin still got emotional when he was around Linda, every time he stopped to think about the close call they had. He had almost lost what he held most dear in his life. Their teenage son became very protective of her, and stuck to her like glue when he was at home. Their 12-year-old daughter grew quiet. Too young to understand much of what went on, their little preschooler was still confused, and just wanted to make sure Mommy didn't leave again.

The one thing no one did, however, was talk about the event. Linda felt some anger, but it was toward the hospital, not Dr. Walker. She knew that accidents did happen. But now that she was a victim, she felt abandoned by the hospital and frustrated that no one there would talk to her about what had happened. This was the same while she was still at the hospital as a patient.

At the same time Linda and her family were trying to navigate through this unfamiliar territory, Jason Walker was feeling lost and abandoned as well. Although Linda had gone home, he still had a powerful desire to communicate with her about the incident. He knew Linda's husband didn't want him to contact her, and the hospital had made their position clear. Without asking the hospital, Jason decided to write her a letter expressing his sorrow and regret for what had happened, taking responsibility and apologizing to Linda. He acknowledged the impact this must have had on her and her family. He also shared with her the impact it had on him, and made sure to let her know he was open to further communication with her. The letter included every possible way Linda could contact him if she wanted to.

Linda received Jason's letter about a week after returning home from the hospital. She dismissed it immediately as nothing more than damage control. Besides, she had bigger things to worry about. Linda's physical recovery and her children took up most of her energy and time. It seemed like worrying about feelings at this point was a luxury she couldn't afford. She knew she couldn't deal with this right now, and filed the letter away.

As she healed physically, Linda's initial euphoria over surviving her ordeal began to wear off. Bombarded with questions from well-meaning friends and neighbors, they often wanted to know if she had seen a bright light when she almost died. And it seemed almost everyone asked her if she was going to sue the doctor and hospital. Even Kevin wanted to file a lawsuit. Linda submerged her feelings in self-defense, and operated on auto-pilot.

Two months after coming home, Linda attended the wake of a child they knew. The tragic nature of the event triggered something deep inside of her. Feelings emerged that Linda hadn't known were there. Once the floodgates opened, the rush of complex emotions was overpowering and paralyzing. She was suddenly aware of how numb she had been during the past weeks.

For the first time since the accident, Linda cried like she would never stop. Why, she wondered, did she get to live, and this child had to die? Guilt over being a survivor haunted Linda as she tried to make sense of the past two months. Whether she wanted to or not, her feelings were here and she couldn't deny them space any longer. Now she would have to deal with them. She desperately wanted to talk about her experiences, but people had moved on and didn't necessarily want to listen. They felt uncomfortable discussing it, and some of them asked outright when she was going to get over this. For them it was in the past, even though she had just begun to feel the impact. She felt like she was going crazy.

A few weeks later Linda met with her orthopedic surgeon, and they began talking about what had happened on the day of her planned surgery three months ago. Her doctor started to explain what that period had been like for him, calling her a miracle, but even with this, he choked up with emotions and had to stop. Seeing his reaction, Linda realized that the incident hadn't just affected her and her family, but it had also affected the healthcare providers who were directly and indirectly involved with her care.

April, 2000

Linda was tired from the runaway emotions and the upheaval the incident had caused in her life. She wanted to address what had happened and regain some control. She wanted her life back. In an effort to seek out support services for patients, she called the hospital to see what was available. Her phone calls went unanswered and she received impersonal, business-like letters from the administration, responses that hit her like a bucket of cold water. It became clear that there was a complete lack of support for patients like her. There were no programs in place to help those who had suffered any kind of avoidable medically induced trauma.

Around this same time, Linda made some decisions for the sake of her sanity. She would not sue the hospital or the doctor. A lawsuit would only drag things out; moreover she and her family had been through enough. Fortunately, aside from the physical scars, there was no other permanent damage. She had been able to return to her normal daily life and activities. In addition, she didn't wish to be responsible for ruining Dr. Walker's career. Linda also decided to face her fears and reschedule surgery. But there was one more thing to resolve. She wanted to speak with Jason Walker, let him know she didn't blame him for the accident, and forgive him so they could both move forward. Thinking they could meet for coffee, she tried calling him, but could not reach him. Jason had moved to San Diego.

Six months after the accident, he received word from a former colleague that Linda was trying to reach him. He wondered why she was contacting him now after so many months, and wondered if this meant she was choosing to take legal action. Although he was apprehensive at first, he overcame his reaction and decided to call her. This was something he had sought out in those early days, and he wanted to follow through. Neither one of them knew that this call would be a turning point that would change their lives going forward.

The phone rang three times before a female's voice came on and said "Hello, this is Linda." Jason quickly explained who he was and why he was calling. The first moments of their conversation were awkward and halting, neither one of them knowing what to expect. Jason was able to answer Linda's questions about the event, filling in many of the gaps and details in the story. He talked about the desperate efforts to save her. She found out that the Bupivacaine had inadvertently been injected into small broken blood vessels near the nerves.

As the conversation became more personal, they each shared the emotional impact that the experience had on them. Then Linda did something Jason never expected; she offered him forgiveness, saying it was something she was doing more for herself. She hoped it would allow her to move forward with her life. This simple act of Linda's touched the invisible wounds Jason had carried with him since that day, and healed the guilt and shame he had felt for months. Then they promised to meet in person the next time the opportunity came up.

November, 2001

Over the next year, Linda and Jason communicated once or twice through letters. It wasn't until the fall that the opportunity to meet they had talked about finally presented itself. They agreed to meet in November, nearly two years to the day after the original event. Jason said he could come to her town outside of Boston. She suggested a little café that had just opened close to her house.

The day arrived, and Linda sat in a booth at the back of the café watching for Jason. She picked a position facing the door so she would see him when he came in. The longer she waited, the more she wondered if she'd been stood up. She thought to herself, *why did I do this?* As a last resort, Linda called his cell phone. A cell phone rang on the other side of the café, and she saw a man stand up and come towards her. He was tall with wide shoulders, and although they had seen each other before, she didn't remember what he looked like. His brown eyes peered out from under a baseball cap, emblazoned with the initials of the hospital where he used to work.

All Linda could think was how much courage it must have taken for him to come there. Seeing him again after everything they had both been through, Linda desperately wanted to give Jason a big hug, but sensed hugging didn't come naturally for him. Reluctantly, she held back from showing her joy and enthusiasm in the way she would with other friends. She'd have to be content with broad smiles and warm handshakes.

They sat in the booth and talked and ate, and at some point, Jason realized that they were no longer a physician and a patient, but people. He went over the technical aspects of what had happened, and how he had felt afterwards. How the hospital had encouraged him to go on with his work and act as if nothing had happened, discouraging him from any contact with Linda or Kevin. Linda talked about her attempts to find help through the hospital, and the impersonal letters she received. She told him about her visit with the orthopedic surgeon. Both of them had known feelings of isolation, fear and guilt. Neither one of them could find support to help them sort through their emotions. Jason said the entire experience was burned in his brain.

Finally they both had what they had longed for in the immediate aftermath two years ago; they each felt heard and understood. Together they recognized the need for some kind of organized support for patients, families and healthcare providers that are involved in medical trauma. If they were unable to find help, then there must be countless others who also suffer alone, like them. After all, according to recent statistics from the Institute of Medicine (IOM) hundreds of patients daily are the victims of preventable adverse medical events. Jason and Linda recognized a need that wasn't being filled, and were struck by the idea that something bigger than their own healing could come from this meeting.

Then and there, Linda committed to establishing a non-profit organization, one that could provide support to people who have been affected by medically induced trauma. Jason said he would serve as the hospital advocate for change.

June 2002

Months of planning followed, and in June of 2002 their vision became a reality. Medically Induced Trauma Support Services, known as MITSS, was incorporated. The mission of MITSS was established to support healing and restore hope to those who have been negatively affected by a medically induced trauma. They defined medically induced trauma as any unexpected complication due to a medical or surgical procedure, a medical systems error, and/or other circumstances that affect the overall well-being of the patient and/or family member. MITSS goal is to assist affected individuals (patients, families, and professionals) to process adverse medical events in a positive manner in order to move forward both personally and professionally.

Jason and Linda's story shows that in the aftermath of an adverse event, those on both sides of the patient-care provider relationship feel the fallout. The defensive walls of silence and secrecy that institutions often throw up in the wake of these events, only serve to create isolation and frustration for everyone involved. These walls destroy the trust between patients and healthcare professionals, and the painful feelings become a breeding ground for the anger and suspicion that fuel so many lawsuits. In many cases there is a better way, moving forward by finding the support to heal, and acknowledging one another's humanity.

Bupivicaine induced cardiotoxicity was found to be the cause of
Linda's cardiovascular collapse, stopping her heart. The drug is used
as a local anesthetic, often administered through an injection before
ankle, hip or knee replacement surgery (arthroplasty). It also is
commonly injected into surgical wound sites to reduce pain for up to
20 hours after surgery.

When he administered the Bupivicaine, Dr. Walker was extremely
careful to insert the syringe away from any direct blood supply. Each
time he placed the needle into the tissue, he withdrew the plunger to
check for blood return in the syringe, and in this case there was no
blood present. This showed him he was not in a vascular area. Even
though perfect technique was utilized, there was a blood vessel near
the nerve that absorbed the anesthetic which traveled to Linda's heart.

Although Linda's event was a rare complication of anesthesia,
rather than a preventable medical error, the same stages of grief and
loss can occur. In both circumstances, anguish, anger and a feeling
of betrayal associated with the hospital and/or care provider may
follow the event. Trust in healthcare is an assumed right. Hospitals are
supposed to heal and not harm. When a preventable medical error or
an adverse event occurs, there is a violation of this trust that can be
overwhelming.

Similarities and differences exist between people's reactions to a
preventable medical error, versus an unexpected adverse event. In the
case of medical errors, people feel justified in directing their anger
toward the doctor or hospital that caused the error. With unexpected
adverse events, there is often no one to blame.

Some people assumed Linda should be grateful and relieved
because healthcare professionals had saved her life. Feelings of anger
seemed out of place, yet those feelings overwhelmed her, and indeed
they were warranted and valid. There was trauma and a loss of control
in a place where Linda should have been safe from harm.

Especially troubling is the fact that most patients have to continue
to receive healthcare services after an unexpected adverse event,

and can't avoid needed care. Even if they were to go to a different medical facility or healthcare professional, they are treated by the same healthcare system that harmed them in the first place. This can produce feelings of anxiety, fear and mistrust, and affect their health and ability to seek further medical attention in a timely fashion.

Recovery from an unplanned event can be as dramatic and difficult. Without resolution and closure following an incident, mistrust can grow and fester. The feelings of grief must be addressed and acknowledged. Hospitals are not set up for this support. The grief response to medical trauma is not recognized. It is rarely discussed or taught to medical social workers or psychologists. Often, patients who have adverse events happen to them end becoming difficult or angry patients. When this happens, it can make future healthcare experiences worse by creating an adversarial relationship between patients and their healthcare providers. Going forward, it is critical for the healthcare system to start recognizing the role of grief recovery for both preventable medical errors and unexpected adverse events.

PROTECT YOURSELF IN TODAY'S HEALTHCARE SYSTEM

After the meeting in the café, Jason and Linda knew that they needed to go beyond the immediate healing of two people. Linda had survived a near-death experience and felt she was left on earth for a purpose. Jason realized there was little help for professionals like him. They also recognized that lack of such support structures often played a role in pushing individuals affected to seek legal recourse. Following their face-to-face meeting and inside calling, they both became committed to making a change in the system.

Linda Kenney founded MITSS in June 2002. Medically Induced Trauma Support Services, or MITSS, whose mission is "To support healing and restore hope" to patients, families and clinicians who have been affected by an adverse medical event.

MITSS achieves its mission by:
- Creating awareness and education. MITSS has been educating the healthcare community on the unique characteristics of

medical trauma, the broad scope of its impact, and the crucial need for support services through participation in forums, local and national conferences, and through the media.

- Providing direct support services to patients, families and clinicians through educational support groups led by clinical psychologists, for those who have been affected by medical errors or unanticipated outcomes. MITSS also provides support groups for nursing professionals who find themselves at the "sharp end" of an adverse medical event.
- Advocacy for action. They encourage and consult with healthcare institutions in developing infrastructures for clinician peer support systems. They also assist in developing a referral process to the MITSS program for patients and families.
- MITSS purpose is to create awareness, promote open and honest communication, and to provide services to patients, families and clinicians affected by medically induced trauma.
- MITSS vision is for all those involved in a medically induced trauma to have access to support services. They envision a more compassionate, patient-centered healthcare system.

ANESTHESIA SAFETY—A PIONEER IN ADVANCING REDUCTION OF MEDICAL ERRORS IN THE OR

In 1984, the Anesthesia Patient Safety Foundation (APSF) was established. The organization has implemented multiple practices to standardize and improve safety for surgical and procedural patients undergoing anesthesia. APSF has a clear mission: "This organization's mission is to ensure that no patient shall be harmed by anesthesia."

The practices promoted by APSF include:
- Protocols for safe anesthesia procedures
- Standardization of anesthesia equipment
- Safety practice standards
- Simulation training in airway management
- Advancing the knowledge base for practitioners of anesthesia

Long before the Institute of Medicine's (IOM) 1999 report, the focus at many of the APSF national and international anesthesiology conferences was on patient safety issues in the operating room (OR). Back in 1989, the practice of anesthesiology began the use of tutorials on patient safety. Tutorials for new anesthesiology residents included such topics as pre-anesthetic evaluation and medication, airway management and endo-tracheal intubation, and intra-operative monitoring. Today, anesthesia care is one of the safest components of healthcare.

When undergoing anesthesia of any type (general, epidural or local), it is important to work closely with your anesthesiologist prior to the procedure. Each anesthesiologist develops an anesthesia plan of care for their patient. The more information provided to them, the more comprehensive their plan can be. Some clinics and hospitals provide pre-anesthesia visits or clinics.

If possible, talk to your anesthesiologist by phone or in person prior to your surgery. Tell your anesthesiologist about previous episodes, complications or reactions that you might have had in the past. Inform them of any drug allergy or sensitivity, and be sure to list all medications including prescriptions, over-the-counter drugs, vitamins, minerals, and herbal supplements. Discuss any specific concerns or anxiety you may have regarding anesthesia.

USING STORIES TO DRIVE CHANGE

Two organizations responded positively to Linda Kenney's traumatic event. The APSF held a workshop in 2005, organized by their executive vice president, Jeffrey B. Cooper, bringing together patients, families and physicians who had experienced an adverse anesthesia event. Dr. Cooper stressed that this is the human side of the equation in anesthesia care, a balance to the remarkable technologic and behavioral progress in the science of patient safety.

A key goal of the program was to introduce a new perspective for the APSF that would be driven by the power of patients and their stories. Dr. Cooper noted that this program was an attempt to open up the filters that physicians often automatically apply to patients' views, and to avoid the reflex responses of "that's not how it's done," or "that can't be done," so often applied to ideas from patients and their survivors. He also commented that one of the reasons it had been difficult to assemble a program of this nature was that, fortunately, anesthesia care catastrophes are exceedingly rare, and that open public discussion can be inhibited by medical-legal constraints.

The workshop featured Linda's story presenting to the workshop members. Anesthesiology is one of the first professions to begin bridging the gap between patients and physicians. While the APSF has sought patient input for many years, this was the first time the foundation was able to organize a program reflecting the perspective of patients, or "victims," of injuries from accidents solely related to anesthesia care.

In addition to Linda's story, two other intensely personal stories of tragic anesthesia events were presented. One was the mother of an 11-year-old boy who suffered massive permanent brain damage from an anesthesia accident, and the other was the wife of a 33-year-old marathon runner, who eventually was allowed to die after an anesthesia mishap. According to Dr. Cooper, their stories simultaneously appalled, entranced and galvanized their audience, motivating them to determine what the APSF can do to help heal their wounds and prevent others from experiencing such trauma.

HEALING AND SUPPORT

The initial letter Linda received from the Chief Medical Officer at the hospital was cold and impersonal. After Linda's work with the hospital things began to change. She was working with another patient and the letter sent by the hospital was entirely opposite of hers and displayed genuine concern and compassion. Linda thought how she would have appreciated a letter like this at the time of her event. The Boston Hospital has now stepped up its efforts to provide support to families. There are support groups for cancer survivors, but little was in place for survivors of traumatic medical events. The Boston hospital has partnered with MITSS to provide links for patients. The hospital now trains their social workers and psychologists in these specialty support services.

Recovery and resolution following medical errors and adverse events still have a long way to go. These concepts are new to the healthcare world, and are evolving following the realization that medical mishaps are prevalent within healthcare, and their impact is greater than recognized in the past. The more hospital leaders, physicians and professional organizations embrace the revolutionary change of adverse event and error acknowledgment and prevention, the sooner healing will occur within hospitals and provide for a better healthcare system.

Medically Induced Trauma:
- Medically Induced Trauma is an unexpected outcome that occurs during medical or surgical care that negatively impacts the emotional and/or physical well being of the patient and/or family members. Medically Induced Trauma is different from other types of trauma since patients and their families may feel:
  - Isolated, because hospitals often are not set up to provide emotional support beyond the hospital stay.
  - The trust between their caregiver, crucial to recovery, has been breached.
  - Vulnerable, since, in most cases, the patient will need continued care within the same system that harmed them.
- If you or a family member has been impacted by a medically induced trauma, please explore how MITSS can assist you. They are there to support you, any way they can.
  - Log onto Medically Induced Trauma Support Services (MITSS) for more information at: http://www.mitss.org

Anesthesia Safety
- Request to speak with or meet your anesthesiologist before undergoing surgery.
- Make a list of your anesthesia history and share it with the anesthesiologist.
- Tell your anesthesiologist and surgeon about all of your allergies.
- Make a printed list of all medicines, vitamins and herbal supplements you take, and give this to your surgeon and anesthesiologist.
- Ask what type of anesthesia you will be receiving. Write down the name. Whether you tolerate the anesthesia well or not, you will want to remember for future reference.
- For more information on anesthesia safety, please visit the Anesthesia Patient Safety Foundation website at: http://www. apsf.org/

CHAPTER 7

ONE OF THEIR

In this chapter
- Learn why as a female of child bearing age you should request a pregnancy test before receiving any treatments or procedures, *even if you use contraceptives.*
- How radiologists can miss important information on imaging studies.
- Classes of drugs and treatments, and how they affect a developing fetus.
- Weighing the risks and benefits of drugs and treatments during pregnancy.

Why avoiding potentially harmful treatments during pregnancy are important to know?

Women in their childbearing years can run the risk of undergoing procedures or receiving medications and treatments without realizing they are pregnant, even if they are using a reliable form of birth control. Common tests and drugs, like x-rays and some antibiotics, can cause birth defects or damage to a developing fetus. Unfortunately, not all hospitals or physicians automatically perform pregnancy tests on female patients when there is a slight possibility of pregnancy or the presence of suspicious symptoms.

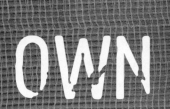

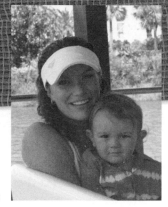

Liz and Ryan

Liz watched Danny, her boyfriend, walk over to the window in their little hut and peer out at the weather as if he could will it to change. The seemingly never-ending rain continued to pelt the glass, as it had almost everyday since they arrived in Fiji over two weeks ago. Palm trees bowed, yielding to the wind, and clouds obscured the island hills in the distance.

This was their last day in paradise. August wasn't supposed to be the rainy season here, at least according to the travel website they used to book the trip. Unfortunately most of their outdoor plans for the week had dissolved in the falling rain. Still, Liz thought as her eyes followed Danny, she was glad they came. Although there hadn't been much snorkeling and surfing it had been a wonderful, romantic get-away, a time to leave work behind and focus on one another. Who cared if it was soggy?

They had first met several years ago, on the job in the emergency room. At the time Liz was a trauma nurse at a Los Angeles area hospital, and Danny was a fire fighter-paramedic who would show up there on calls periodically. Both of them were involved with other people back then, but even so, Danny half-jokingly told a co-worker that he thought Liz was beautiful and he wanted to marry her someday. Slim and athletic, Liz was an accomplished skier, horsewoman and cyclist, with a curly cascade of light brunette hair. Danny had broad shoulders and a muscular build, and his dark brown eyes appeared to smile along with his mouth. Liz thought he was gorgeous but believed that firefighters were trouble, better at flirting than long-term relationships, so she kept her distance. Besides, he was a bit cocky.

It wasn't until years later, in March of 2002, that the two of them connected. Liz was at a conference on emergency medicine at a mountain resort area, and Danny happened to be at the same location snowboarding with a fellow firefighter. Neither one of them was seeing anyone special. At first she tried to set him up with another nurse who was a friend, but there was an unmistakable attraction between Liz and Danny, and they became inseparable during the trip. They would ski the most difficult slopes together, and he was impressed she could keep up with him. When they would finally tire, they sat among the trees in the snow and talked for hours. By the end of the trip they both knew this could be "it." That was five months ago. They had agreed to take things slowly.

Now it was time to leave the island paradise to return to the real world, and reluctantly they packed for their trip back to L.A. This was a demanding time in Liz's life. Just 29 years old, currently she helped to oversee the quality of care and compliance with regulations for the six Los Angeles County hospitals. Patient safety was a professional passion for Liz. She felt like she was really making a difference and affecting the care of a greater number of patients through her work. And as if life wasn't busy enough, she was completing her master's degree in nursing. She knew she would have to hit the ground running after their trip.

Liz also had a health issue that cropped up just before their vacation to Fiji, one she would need to deal with when she got home. Her blood pressure had recently gone up sharply, and she had blood in her urine. This premature hypertension, high blood pressure at such an early age in an otherwise healthy, fit woman, was a red flag that required attention. Her primary care physician suspected a kidney problem. The doctor started her on medication for hypertension, and they had performed a renal ultrasound on her kidneys at the end of July. It showed diminished blood flow to her kidneys, and she would need to see a nephrologist, or kidney specialist, as well as an urologist.

After the Labor Day holiday the doctors ordered another test, an MRA, or magnetic resonance angiogram, a type of MRI that provides images of blood flow and shows the condition of blood vessels. This would give them a clearer picture of what was going on in the kidneys. Liz' MRA showed evidence of fibromuscular dysplasia, or FMD. It looked much like a string of pearls in her kidneys. The condition can cause renal stenosis, a dangerous narrowing of the renal arteries, the major blood vessels in the kidneys. That would account for her high blood pressure and the blood in her urine.

Liz began researching FMD, visiting online health groups and reading everything she could find on the disease. Although she was a nurse, the Internet provided a portal to hard-to-find information and a network of other people who either knew about the condition, or suffered from it themselves. The more obscure your disease, the more important these resources could be.

By accessing research and information, Liz discovered FMD was connected to an inherited condition found in her background. Her family medical history included an unusual connective tissue disorder, Ehler-Danlos syndrome, that can cause vascular problems in some affected people, and her grandmother had died from an aneurysm as a result of the disorder.

The dysplasia, or abnormal cell development caused by FMD, often involves the walls of one or more arteries in the body, and is most commonly found in the renal arteries. Researchers have found a family link but no known cause for the disease, which affects more women than men. The most favored treatment is renal angioplasty, a balloon procedure on the blood vessels in the kidneys. Liz' urologist scheduled the procedure for October 18.

As the weeks of September passed, Liz felt unusually tired. Running and working out normally gave her an energy boost, but now she just felt drained after exercising. Since she had always been active and healthy this concerned her. She assumed it was the result of her elevated blood pressure and the medication she was taking for it. Her blood pressure kept gradually getting higher and higher. At one point in late September, Liz had blurry vision and headaches. When she took her own blood pressure at home, she discovered it was 198 over 110, a dangerous level. Afraid of missing work, she took an extra blood pressure pill to compensate for the rise and it went down.

While waiting for the angioplasty in mid-October, Liz realized she never had a regular period at the end of September, only spotting. Because of everything going on in her life, she didn't think much about it at the time. Skipped periods and spotting were not uncommon on birth control pills, and the additional stress and health-related problems also could easily affect things. Although she was taking oral contraceptives, she bought a home pregnancy test just as a precaution. Home tests had become more reliable in recent years, so she was relieved when the results were negative.

Danny came with Liz on the day of the procedure, and patiently waited. A nurse asked Liz when her last menstrual period was as they prepared her for the angioplasty. Liz told her she was a couple of weeks late. They began giving her a combination of medications to make the experience more tolerable, including the anesthesia drug Fentanyl, and Versed, a narcotic for pain. Liz was in a relaxed and dreamy state, awake and aware, but altered. The radiologist, Dr. Marvin inserted a line into the femoral artery on the right side of her groin.

Dr. Marvin began by injecting nitroglycerin to dilate the artery, followed by heparin to prevent the blood from clotting. He deftly performed the balloon dilation on the right side first, before moving on to the left side. There was no comparison in the pain. Even with the sedative effects of the drugs, the discomfort on the left side was excruciating. Dr. Marvin continued, giving her more heparin and using a larger balloon. She begged the doctor to stop. He seemed relatively unconcerned about the level of pain she was experiencing and continued.

At the end of the procedure they were unable to remove the femoral line because her blood clotting levels were abnormal, putting Liz at risk for excessive bleeding, likely from the large doses of heparin. She was placed in the intensive care unit overnight. Her pain was so intense that it caused vomiting. The radiologist still didn't seem to recognize the severity of Liz's pain and refused to give her morphine, prescribing Vicodin instead, but it was ineffective because she was unable to keep it down. At that point, Danny had watched Liz suffer for too long and he demanded that the nurses get an order for morphine to ease her pain so she could sleep.

By morning, Liz' clotting levels had retreated to normal and the doctor was able to take out the line. A huge knot had formed by her groin, a grossly swollen bruise that was a souvenir from the arterial line. Liz agreed to go to Danny's house, where he could keep an eye on her and she would have someone to help for a few days. But the pain and vomiting continued after her release, and Liz called the urologist.

On Monday Danny took her back to the hospital, where a doctor ordered an abdominal CT scan. The scan showed an area of dead tissue in her left kidney, called a cortical infarct. It appeared that the angioplasty balloon the urologist used was too big and it had torn a section of her left renal artery, producing a large clot and the terrible pain she had experienced and damage to the kidney tissue. She was told the injured portion of the kidney would not heal completely, but would still function.

While her recovery took longer than she would have liked, Liz eventually returned to her normal schedule at work and school. She was almost done with classes, and would soon have her master's degree. Her blood pressure was controlled with medication. Although she still had nausea and some fatigue, she continued to assume it was due to her blood pressure or the prescriptions she was taking.

In December Liz began looking for a starter house to buy, the fulfillment of a dream to own a little place of her own. She found a quaint two-bedroom bungalow nestled in Westchester. Although it was small, it was in a beautiful well-established neighborhood, and even had a yard—a rare commodity in any LA neighborhood.

That same month, Liz paid a visit to the nurse practitioner at her gynecologist's office. She had gained five pounds, despite watching what she ate and exercising, and she felt bloated and puffy. Her energy level was still lagging and she wasn't menstruating. Liz told the nurse about the negative home pregnancy test she used earlier, as well as all of the medical complications and stress she'd endured over the past few months. The nurse practitioner agreed that a multitude of things could cause missed periods, including stress, heavy exercise and hormone imbalances. She suggested a progesterone-only birth control pill.

As 2002 came to a close, the doctors took Liz off of her medications. Her blood pressure had retreated to normal levels and she felt better, but was still tired much of the time. She wasn't herself, and Danny was angry that more had not been done to get to the bottom of Liz' symptoms. His intuition as a healthcare professional made him think there was more to her condition than was previously thought.

Liz and Danny rang in 2003 at a big party with friends, toasting the New Year with drinks, and hoping the health problems were behind them. This was a time to celebrate. Liz and Danny were in love and had each other, Liz had just bought her first home, and she was finally starting her last semester of graduate school.

Several days later, when Liz crawled into bed one night, she tried to roll onto her stomach and something stopped her cold. She felt a ball in her lower abdomen, a large, firm mass that prevented her from rolling over. Gripped by fear over what health crisis might be next, her imagination ran wild with images of ovarian tumors or serious kidney complications. And although she dreaded more bad news, she was anxious to find out what was wrong and called the doctor as soon as possible.

Flat on her back on the examining table, Liz lay there impatiently, wondering what the doctor suspected as she prodded Liz' abdomen. All of the frightening possibilities came to mind as she lay there. It was January 22, months after her health issues had surfaced. The gynecologist explained that, indeed, he had found something, but probably not what Liz was expecting—and expecting was the operative word. She was pregnant. Liz held her breath and her jaw went slack with surprise. Her doctor slipped out of the examining room for a few moments and returned with a Doppler ultrasound.

As the sensor slid over the cold, wet gel on her belly, Liz heard the clear, rhythmic swoosh-swoosh of a baby's heartbeat. Initially the gynecologist said it looked like she was about 18 weeks along, but on further examination and testing they learned it was closer to 22 weeks. Stunned didn't begin to describe how Liz felt; she felt more like she had been hit by lightening. Of all the scenarios she pictured, this was never one she considered. How did a person get used to the idea of walking in to a doctor's office not pregnant, and minutes later walking out more than halfway to their due date? The home test had been negative, and none of the doctors who treated her mentioned anything about pregnancy. Her brain was in overdrive, trying to process all of the images and consequences.

Now so many of her symptoms made sense in the context of this new information: the missed periods, the terrible nausea, the weight gain and bloating, the extreme fatigue. It wasn't the fibromuscular dysplasia at all. The doctors all were so focused on her FMD that they had missed the obvious warning signs of another condition, even with the multiple x-ray and MRI images they read. Surely something must have shown up.

Liz thought back to the Fiji Islands in August, and their romantic holiday in the tropical rain. She thought of Danny. Danny! How would she tell him? They'd been together for a year, and after her stay in the ICU Danny had told her that it made him realize how important she was to him. He said he knew he wanted to spend the rest of his life with her, but they hadn't made any formal plans yet. What would he think of this?

Then the most horrifying thoughts of all, the long list of procedures she'd had, of drugs they put into her body while her baby was growing. The MRA, the abdominal x-rays, the CT scan, the angioplasty with the contrast dye, the narcotics and anesthesia, blood thinners and blood pressure medication. Even though she tried to block the thoughts, fleeting images of deformed and disabled children crowded into her head uninvited. What if her baby had suffered irreparable harm?

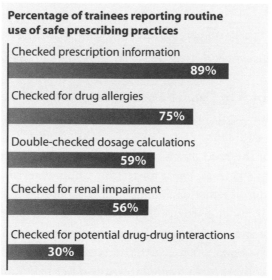

Source: Garbutt JM, Highstein G, Jeffe DB, Dunagan WC, Praser VJ.
Safe medication prescribing: training and experience of medical students
and house staff at a large teaching hospital. Acad Med. 2005; 80: 594-599.

Liz kept her composure as she quickly made her way to her car, and managed to get inside before breaking down and sobbing, resting her head against the steering wheel. She sat in the driver's seat of the parked car and phoned Danny from her cell phone, begging him to come home.

"Please Danny!" she pleaded. "You have to come home right away."

"I can't leave the station. There's no one to cover for me. Are you alright? Are you hurt?" He started asking questions, fearing she'd been in an accident or had a serious medical crisis. "Just tell me what's wrong." He could hear her crying uncontrollably and it frightened him.

Liz was terrified of Danny's reaction. She couldn't tell him over the phone like this. But she had no choice.

"I'm pregnant," she blurted out through her tears, nearly choking as she tried to calm down and breathe normally again. There was only silence at the other end of the line, and Liz didn't know what to make of it.

After several seconds that seemed more like several minutes, Danny spoke. "How far along are you?"

"Over five months." Even as she said it, Liz still couldn't quite believe it.

"It's okay, really. This is great." He sounded excited. "In fact, this is fantastic!" he said enthusiastically. "Everything's going to be fine. It's alright."

Liz was elated by Danny's reaction, and reassured by his calm insistence that everything would be fine. She could handle anything if he was in this with her.

Because of the procedures and drugs during the pregnancy, Liz was referred to a perinatologist for testing. She was terribly worried over the amount of radiation and medications the baby had been exposed to. Liz felt angry that no one had performed a basic serum pregnancy test as a routine part of the screening process. It was obvious that the home pregnancy test was either incorrect or done too early. At this point she just wanted to know if her baby was alright. While there was nothing she could do about it if something was wrong, at least she and Danny could prepare themselves. They started reading everything they could find on the Internet about x-ray and drug exposure during pregnancy.

During a full three-dimensional ultrasound, Liz searched the monitor looking for the baby's outline. The image appeared to be normal, but she was especially eager to see the fingers. Because of the radiation, she was afraid their baby might have flippers instead, so she insisted the technician focus on the tiny hands. To their relief, the ultrasound showed a perfectly-shaped baby boy with all the right parts, but a little small for his gestational age. After all, Liz didn't know she was eating for two, and had only gained ten pounds. She would need to eat more to help the baby catch up. The only other abnormalities seemed to be diminished amniotic fluid and a placenta that was smaller than normal. Liz saw Danny cry for the first time, overjoyed that the baby seemed to be alright.

Wanting to determine everything her baby had been exposed to, Liz obtained her medical records from all the tests and procedures. She was shocked to discover her CT scan showed a mass. None of her doctors who saw the results had questioned what the mass might be, and yet it was clearly visible on the imaging. Not even the radiologist questioned it. Liz was appalled. That mass was her baby! She could have, should have, known back in October. Now they could only wait to see if their unborn child had been damaged.

Deep in her gut, Liz had a dark, hidden fear and secretly waited for something to go wrong. She felt powerless, not knowing whether her baby had been affected. Furious with the four doctors who had treated her, she contacted each one in late January to tell them about the baby. Her primary care doctor had a particularly chilling reaction to the news; he said he was thankful he wasn't the one to order the angioplasty, because that meant he wouldn't be "named in a lawsuit." When she questioned the nephrologist about how he could have missed the mass, he told her he only read the part involving her kidney.

For the next four months, Danny and Liz hung on to every ultrasound that appeared normal, every positive test result. Twice a week Liz went to the doctor's office so they could measure the amniotic fluid. By now, she had a new gynecologist who wanted to induce her labor at the end of May, but before that could happen Liz went into labor on her own, and on May 28, 2003, their son Ryan was born. Small at six pounds, one ounce, he was nonetheless healthy and perfect, the spitting image of Danny. And although he showed no ill effects from everything he had been through, as a precaution Danny and Liz arranged to freeze his cord blood, just in case there were health issues that cropped up later. They looked at it as added insurance.

After Ryan's birth, Liz met with the hospital's risk manager. She was polite and apologetic, but what Liz wanted was action. She wanted pregnancy tests to be a routine part of the intake process for women in their childbearing years, and asked to meet with the hospital again after two months so they could update her on what they had done to correct the situation. She also wrote a letter to The Joint Commission shortly before the hospital was up for review, and they cited the hospital for lack of communication.

Danny and Liz are happily married, and Ryan is, in Liz' words, "too bright for his own good." He is very much his parents' child, sharp witted and athletic, with a love of the outdoors. Since his birth their family has grown. Ryan now has a younger brother, Evan. Liz and Danny still travel to exotic locations with the children.

Liz continues to work in patient safety. Looking back on what happened to her, she is acutely aware of the irony that, although she works with issues of healthcare quality and risk management, she was the victim of a potentially devastating medical error. "I *was in* the system," she says. "If it could happen to me, it could happen to anyone."

Coming out of her experience, her hope is that healthcare professionals won't assume other healthcare providers don't have the same needs that other patients do. But most of all, Liz would like all healthcare professionals to "Listen to the patient."

Her advice to patients is even more direct. "Don't be afraid to make enemies. You're not there to make friends; you're there for your health. Stand up. Get loud. Get mean. Take charge! Do whatever it takes."

Despite being a registered nurse, and working in the field of quality improvement, patient safety and risk management, Liz experienced a medical error. Liz had the following procedures and drugs during the early stages of her unborn baby's development: abdominal CT, MRA, renal angioplasty with radiographic imaging (x-ray), contrast dye, arterial line insertion, Heparin, Nitroglycerine, Versed, Fentanyl, Morphine Sulfate, Vicodin, various blood pressure medications and oral contraceptives.

A magnetic resonance angiogram (MRA) uses a magnetic field and pulses of radio wave energy to create pictures of blood vessels inside the body. It is a type of magnetic resonance imaging (MRI). An MRA can detect problems with the blood vessels that may be causing reduced blood flow. The test is often used to evaluate the blood vessels leading to the brain, legs or kidneys, as in this case. In most instances, this test is not recommended during the first trimester of pregnancy.

Liz' CT scan showed endometrial density suggestive of pregnancy. Four physicians viewed the CT scan results, including her radiologist, urologist, nephrologist and primary care physician. Although the radiologist recommended an ultrasound, no additional diagnostic tests to detect pregnancy were ever ordered and completed, such as a serum (blood) pregnancy test.

While the primary care physician was unapologetic, and simply glad he couldn't be targeted for litigation, the nephrologists was much more contrite and said that the finding should have been questioned. However, ultimately the radiologist is the physician who is responsible for interpreting the imaging results. In the end, Liz did not take legal action against any of the healthcare providers involved.

Investigating the mass and determining there was a pregnancy most likely would have altered Liz' course of treatment. Missing the obvious on radiology imaging is more common than many people may realize. Physicians, including radiologists, occasionally become focused on one result, neglecting to pursue alternative possibilities. Imaging shadows may be mistaken for something other than what they are.

Nonetheless, there were many other opportunities for physicians to order a serum pregnancy test, especially considering Liz' age and missed menstrual periods. A precautionary pregnancy test was certainly indicated. Although Liz had used a home pregnancy test, the physicians should not have assumed that it was accurate, or that it replaced the need for a controlled laboratory test.

Liz received multiple medications during the course of her treatment, and no doubt many of these drugs would not have been used if the doctors knew about her pregnancy. Medications are rated by the U.S. Food and Drug Administration (FDA) into categories of safety for pregnant women, designed to guide physicians in the dispensing of necessary medications for this group of patients. Many medications are considered safe for the developing fetus, but others pose a significant risk, and should not be dispensed during pregnancy. The FDA labeled categories for pregnant women include A, B, C, D and X.

Category A:
- Adequate and well-controlled studies have failed to demonstrate risk on the fetus.
- Possibility of fetal harm appears remote.

Category B:
- Controlled Studies done on animals in reproduction do not indicate risk to the fetus.
- No adequate and well-controlled studies done on pregnant women.

Category C:
- Studies on animals show adverse effect and toxicity on fetus.
- No adequate and well-controlled studies have been done on pregnant women.
- Drugs should be given only if the potential benefit outweighs the potential fetal risk.

Category D:
- Positive evidence of human fetal risk exists.
- Potential benefits may warrant use of the drug in pregnant women despite potential risks (e.g. life threatening situations or serious illness).

Category X:
- Positive evidence of human fetal risk exists.
- Potential benefits may warrant use of the drug in pregnant women despite potential risks (e.g. life threatening situations or serious illness).
- Studies in animals and/or humans have demonstrated fetal abnormalities.
- Fetal risk involved in use of drug clearly outweighs potential benefit.
- Contraindicated in women who are or may become pregnant.
- Don't use.

The medications administered to Liz during the course of her treatment fell into the following categories:
- Heparin: Category B
- Vicodin: Category B, unless used for extended time and in high doses at full term pregnancy. Then the drug is rated category D
- Morphine Sulfate: Category B, same as above for term pregnancy
- Fentanyl: Category B
- Norvasc: Category C
- Nitroglycerine products: Category C
- Versed: Category D
- Oral Contraceptives: Category X
- X-ray exposure with contrast dye: Not recommended in the first trimester of pregnancy

Critically important, aside from category C, D and X medications, is that none of these drug combinations have been studied together to know their collective impact on a developing fetus. Liz was a healthy 29-year-old, and normally her body could handle the medications she received. However, if a simple lab test determined her pregnancy status, then the medication regimen could have been immediately adjusted to avoid categories C through X.

PROTECT YOURSELF IN TODAY'S HEALTHCARE SYSTEM

Asking a woman about her menstrual history is a standard question that is built into almost every health assessment form or questionnaire. Some medical questionnaires now require that a physician sign the form to show that the doctor has reviewed the information. With any missed or unusual menstrual period in a woman of childbearing age, a laboratory (blood) pregnancy test should be performed. Although home pregnancy tests can be accurate, they are not as reliable as a simple blood test for the pregnancy hormone, human chorionic gonadotropin (hCG), and they are not considered a replacement for a lab test.

Some women develop an illness or succumb to an injury during pregnancy, and a small amount of radiographic imaging (X-ray) appears safe. The measurement of radiation exposure is composed of high energy photons called grey (Gy) and rem, more commonly known as "rads." Ionizing radiation photons are capable of damaging DNA and generating caustic free radicals that can cause cancer.

Because it is not safe to study high doses of radiation exposure in humans, most data on radiation exposure comes from studies on pregnant women in Nagasaki and Hiroshima, Japan, after the atomic bomb explosions of the 1940s. Among women who were pregnant during that time, 28 percent aborted, 25 percent gave birth to children who died within the first year of life, and 28 percent had children with severe birth defects of the central nervous system. According to an article in the American Family Physician (1999, April 1), radiation effects on the fetus are grouped into three categories: teratogenesis (fetal malformation), carcinogenesis (induced malignancy), and mutagenesis (alteration of genes). According to the same article, the most common fetal malformations caused by high-dose radiation are microcephaly and mental retardation.

Rad exposure varies widely among the type of radiographic studies. For example, it would take 50,000 dental X-rays to equal an exposure of five rads. By contrast, it takes only one abdominal CT scan to equal five rads. Generally, women in Japan were exposed to large doses of rads, from a minimum of ten, to a dose of 150 or greater. Aside from the fetal risk, it takes smaller doses of rad exposure to increase the chance of childhood malignancies in the exposed fetus.

In particular, the incidence of leukemia is slightly higher at 5 per 10,000, versus 3.66 per 10,000 in the general population. This is why Danny and Liz had the baby's cord blood frozen, to be used in treatment in the event that Ryan someday developed leukemia.

Unless absolutely necessary, most imaging studies are delayed until after the first trimester of pregnancy, or in some cases delayed until after the birth of the baby. Most likely, Liz' tests and treatments could have been delayed until after the birth of Ryan, and her blood pressure could have been controlled with an effective regimen of category B medications.

Liz' case represents a need for hospitals and physicians to follow basic rules for sound care. None of the breakdowns in assessment and communication represented here were complicated, or the result of technology issues. Basic screening for pregnancy, closer review of imaging studies and a more thorough history of the patient may have avoided these medical errors. One key principle in error prevention is to slow down and follow the essential steps of patient assessment and diagnostic evaluations. This is the foundation for preventing some of the common adverse events in healthcare.

Pregnancy and your treatment or procedure:

- If you suspect you could be pregnant and are in need of radiographic tests, a new medication or a medical procedure, ask a physician to perform a serum (blood) pregnancy test first.
- If you are pregnant and are prescribed medication(s) by a physician, learn the FDA category for each medication.
  - Discuss with your doctor the risks and benefits of any medication that is prescribed to you.
- Complete all medical forms and questionnaires thoroughly.
  - Ask your physician to review the forms, and make sure you point out any section that highlights a significant history, condition, illness or injury.

Additional tips when going for X-Rays:

- Occasionally, a woman may mistake the symptoms of pregnancy for the symptoms of a disease:
  - If you have any of the symptoms of pregnancy—nausea, vomiting, breast tenderness, fatigue, bloating, missed menstrual cycle(s)—consider whether you might be pregnant and tell your doctor or x-ray technologist before having any x-ray. A laboratory pregnancy test may be needed.
- If you ARE pregnant or think you might be, and are asked to hold a child for him/her to be x-rayed, decline and explain that you are or might be pregnant.
- If you are NOT pregnant and you are asked to hold a child during an x-ray, be sure to ask for a lead apron to protect your reproductive organs.
- Whenever an x-ray is requested, tell your doctor about any similar x-rays you might have had in the recent past. It may not be necessary to do another.
- It is a good to keep a record of the x-ray examinations you and

your family have had taken so you can provide this kind of information accurately.

Feel free to talk with your doctor about the need for an x-ray examination. You should understand the reason x-rays are requested in your particular case.

THEY'RE NOT

In this chapter

- Understand what measures you can take if you or a family member is receiving inadequate emergency care.
- Find out why communication is vital to a correct diagnosis, and how physician tunnel vision undermines it.
- Learn the importance of knowing where to get emergency help or where the code blue button is when you are alone with a patient in a hospital emergency examining room.
- Know the signs of an aortic aneurysm.

Why not getting the proper attention and care in the ED can matter to you?

Many of the nation's hospital emergency departments are crowded or understaffed. Long waiting times and poor communication with healthcare professionals are all too common. Studies indicate many physicians make up their minds about a patient's ailment and condition in the first 18 seconds they see them. It can be difficult for a patient or family member to make doctors listen and keep an open mind after that point. As a result, healthcare professionals may miss critical signs and symptoms that could save a life.

LISTENING

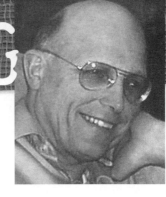

Ken Simon

It was 9:00 a.m., July 12, 2003, a glorious Saturday morning on what promised to be a hot day, at least by the standards of Snohomish, Washington. Nestled in a valley halfway between Puget Sound to the west and the Cascade mountains on the east, the climate was usually mild and often moist, and hot was a relative term.

Jennifer Simon was in the field with the horses after breakfast, behind the cozy little house she called their cottage. In the distance she could see the back deck where they had just eaten. Now her husband Ken was out there, drenched in sunlight, doing his morning yoga and meditation. Steam was rising off the roof as the nighttime dew evaporated in the rising heat. She could hear the hawks, and looking up she spotted one soaring overhead. It was a pastoral scene, so peaceful. As she walked in the opposite direction of the house, she gazed back over her shoulder at Ken one more time and thought how lucky they were to live there.

Ken and Jennifer Simon lived in the Snohomish Valley in a small, comfortable home they had bought in 1974, just a few years after they had gotten married. They had raised their two children on this tranquil five-acre farm, an idyllic setting where Jennifer trained horses and the kids were involved in 4-H Club.

A few things had changed over the years, of course. They remodeled the house and raised it up on pilings after the big Northwest floods of 1996, in an effort to avoid more damage in the future. Both the children were grown now. Their son, Mark, was 26, living and working in Seattle, and dating a physician. Monique, their 24-year-old daughter, loved the outdoors and was on her way to a backwoods adventure in the Alaskan wilderness. But the farm held memories and a quiet permanence for Ken and Jennifer, and they never wanted to leave. Now they lived there with two horses and their dog, Buck, an enormous, lovable 120-pound black lab.

Jennifer still trained horses, as well as repairing saddles and horse tack for some of her clients, and she was formerly a veterinary assistant. Ken had always worked in aviation, and flying was his passion as far back as high school. At the age of 18, he took flying lessons at a small, private airfield in the area, and Jennifer would sit and wait for him in the airport ground school. Later he obtained his instrument rating so he could fly more complex aircraft. During his career Ken had been a flight instructor, a pilot and flight captain for Horizon Air, worked on safety for Boeing, and spent 16 years in the Federal Aviation Administration (FAA) rising through the ranks. He had more than 10,000 hours of flight time as a pilot in command. Along the way, he taught his son and his own father to fly.

Most recently Ken had worked as the primary operations inspector for Alaska Airlines 737 program. As a part of his work, his zeal and enthusiasm for safety motivated him to complete one of his most important professional projects, one about which he felt very strongly.

Ken had long thought that emergency procedures should be available in writing for pilots, and reviewed along with other checklists before every commercial flight. Although pilots must have these procedures committed to memory, a commercial pilot rarely encounters an emergency, and he argued that relying on memory at a critical time was not enough. In spite of resistance from some in the airline industry, Ken aggressively pushed the project through because it would make passengers and crew safer. He oversaw the creation and implementation of a written emergency checklist to be completed along with every preflight checklist throughout Alaska Airlines, and he was rewarded by the industry for his efforts. In May of 2003, he received the FAA's award for safety inspector of the year in his region.

After tending the animals that Saturday, Jennifer returned to the house and found Ken at his computer, doing some research and balancing his checking account. She smiled as she looked at him from behind. They'd been together forever it seemed, meeting back in the 60s when they were in high school, then marrying several years later in 1970. More than 32 years later, Ken was still a good-looking, athletic man. Lean and 6 feet tall, he had soft blue-gray eyes and constantly smiled. Jennifer thought that if he had any fault at all, it was being too kind.

Like many men his age, Ken had some cardiovascular issues. Now 55 years old, he had well-controlled high blood pressure, and a slightly enlarged heart from an aortic valve insufficiency, a defect in the way the valve performed. But he was under the care of a cardiologist, and he was fanatical about his diet and exercise regimen. He did yoga every morning, ran six to ten miles daily, ate healthy foods and monitored his blood pressure daily. In fact, Ken was in such great shape that his cardiologist cleared him to run marathons.

July 12, 12:00 Noon
It was getting near lunchtime, and the Simons began to discuss plans for what they would do that afternoon. They were briefly interrupted by one of Jennifer's friends, who stopped by to talk about 4-H and drop off a book about Seabiscuit, the legendary racehorse. Alone once again, Jennifer sat leafing through the borrowed book and Ken looked at the movies playing nearby. They decided to see *Pirates of the Caribbean* after lunch. With their decision made, Ken stood up and headed for the kitchen.

Just seconds after he left the room, she heard Ken cry out from the kitchen, yelling her name frantically. "Jennifer! Jennifer!"

She let the book fall to the floor and ran the 20 feet to the kitchen doorway, dodging furniture. She saw Ken staggering backward, clutching the center of his chest with his hands. He looked white as a ghost. Standing in front of him, she tried to guide him back into a kitchen chair but he was missing it. Ken was so much bigger than she was. Jennifer grabbed his upper arms just above the elbow and pivoted his body, easing him down to the bare floor.

Jennifer asked him if she should call for an ambulance, then realized he couldn't speak at all. She knew he was in serious trouble, and thought maybe it was a heart attack. Kneeling down by Ken, she held his hands for a few seconds and felt how icy they were. After dialing 9-1-1, Jennifer ran and snatched a pillow off the couch, fearing he would hurt his head lying on the hard kitchen floor. It seemed silly later, but at the time she didn't want him to be uncomfortable.

When she went back to Ken, he was talking again, saying "Take my blood pressure." She placed the pillow under his head and left to get his blood pressure cuff. Lowering herself back to the floor, Jennifer wrapped the cuff around his arm and began to take his pressure. It didn't look right. She couldn't get a reading, and didn't know if was due to Ken's condition or if she wasn't using the equipment correctly. *I should have used it more often*, she thought. Ken always took his own blood pressure; she never had to do it.

Five minutes had gone by—an eternity. Time had taken on new dimensions. At last she heard the approaching sirens, and decided she should put their dog in the bedroom so he wouldn't interfere. Rising from the floor one more time, she dragged a reluctant Buck by his collar and shoved him into their room, slamming the door behind him.

Carrying a gurney up the flight of stairs to the front door, the medics knocked. As Jennifer opened the door, one of the medics said something about having the wrong clipboard. They entered the house, and one of them began asking Ken questions as they gave him an aspirin to chew and started an IV line. Ken could talk to them, but not in complete sentences. He mumbled in short, clipped phrases describing his symptoms. "Telescoping vision. Dizzy. Tingling hands. Chest pain." Using two fingers, he pointed to the middle of his chest. He said the pain was like a punch in the sternum, the worst pain he ever had. Asked to rate his pain on a scale of 10, he said it was "Ten out of 10."

The medics went back and forth among themselves about the best way to get Ken out of the house and down to the ambulance. They didn't think they could get him out the front door and down the stairs on the gurney, so they tried standing him up. He staggered and began to fall, and they realized it wouldn't work. Eventually they made the decision to take him out the back way, from the elevated deck. Jennifer wished they could have figured it out more quickly.

She asked the paramedics where they were taking him, and after they loaded Ken into the ambulance she jumped in her truck to follow. They sat there in the driveway for a long time, and she wondered what on Earth they were doing. Finally they pulled out and headed for the hospital, no lights or sirens in use. Jennifer kept close behind them for the trip to the local hospital.

Three blocks from the hospital the ambulance ran a red light, and Jennifer kept on going with them. A police car she hadn't noticed came up behind her with flashing lights, and tried to pull her over. She stopped briefly, but drove off without permission, explaining to the officer that her husband was in the ambulance. The police officer was skeptical, and followed her to the hospital to make sure she was telling the truth. *Now they had gotten there ahead of her,* Jennifer worried.

July 12, 1:00 P.M.

As Jennifer entered the emergency department, police officer in tow, the paramedics were just bringing Ken in on the gurney. They were met by the triage team, the staff that would assess his condition and start his care. As they took him to the first room on the right, room 12, she heard the medics calling out their report on his condition.

"He LOC'd on us three times," they said. Jennifer knew *LOC* meant *loss of consciousness.* This had occurred during a 15 minute ride. "BP is 80 over palp," the paramedics continued. *Palp,* was shorthand for palpable, indicating that no real number registered. His blood pressure was 80 over some number so small that it was insignificant. What did it all mean? Something was terribly wrong.

A triage nurse began asking Ken questions. He was conscious now, but couldn't really talk except to say single words. "Heavy. Sharp. Throbbing," he kept repeating, as he continued to point at his chest. "Ten out of 10," he told them with difficulty, just as he told the paramedics before.

Jennifer could tell that Ken was frightened by his own confusion, and that made her feel all the more panicked. He was her rock. As a pilot, he was the one who always kept his cool no matter what was going on around him. It was part of his nature as well as his training. She remembered one time when just the two of them were flying, and Ken was at the controls. An engine stalled out, and she silently watched her husband as he handled the situation. Remaining calm and quiet, Ken methodically brought the plane back under control and landed it safely. But now he was uncertain and bewildered, and he seemed to feel an impending sense of doom.

Still white as a sheet, Ken suddenly and unexpectedly spoke an entire sentence with total clarity. "My vision telescoped, like a jet pilot that's taken too many Gs." Jennifer was surprised he was so lucid, but he was in intense pain.

Taking his hands in hers to reassure him, she again felt the coldness. The odd thing was that his hands and feet were usually the warmest of anyone's. He had a high metabolism, and she often joked that he was her "pot bellied stove," capable of keeping her warm under the coldest conditions. He complained one more time that his hands and feet were tingly.

They hooked Ken up to a cardiac monitor, applying a second set of electrodes to add to the ones the paramedics had used, and Jennifer could see the digital readout of his heart rate—over 200 beats per minute. He said his chest felt heavy and tight.

More questions were asked in an effort to gauge his mental state. "What year is it? Who is the president?" a nurse asked. Ken didn't know where he was, and for some reason he thought the year was 1998. The only thing he knew for certain was Jennifer's name and his own. He was scared when he didn't know things, and she was scared for him.

July 12, 1:20 P.M.

It had been a good 15 or 20 minutes since they arrived, and no doctor had entered to check on Ken. Behind a curtain in the same examining area, Jennifer could hear a conversation between a physician and a female patient. The doctor was casually talking about where the patient's follow-up care would take place, and all the while Jennifer was wondering why the doctor wasn't coming to see her husband.

Another few minutes passed before a young, ordinary-looking man entered the room. He planted himself in a chair at the foot of Ken's bed, slouching in his seat looking disinterested and preoccupied. He never introduced himself, but they assumed by his questions that he was the emergency physician. He asked the same questions that others had already asked Ken, and he said he would order tests to determine if Ken was having a heart attack. Ken seemed agitated by the doctor's questions and anxious because he couldn't remember things.

"I can't find the words," he told the doctor. "Ask her; she knows the answers," he said, looking over at his wife. Jennifer only wished she had all the answers.

She explained that Ken was under the care of a cardiologist at a local clinic, and told the ER doctor about his aortic valve insufficiency and high blood pressure. But she let him know that her husband's hypertension was very well-controlled with a half-tablet of medication, and that lately his average blood pressure had been running 120 over 60, better than many who were younger or fitter. The ER doctor talked. But the doctor never touched or examined Ken, even to listen to his heart with a stethoscope.

July 12, 2:00 P.M.

By 2:00 Ken's speech was beginning to improve, yet his pulse rate was still erratic, fluctuating up to 200 beats-per-minute although he was just lying still in a bed. Jennifer was sure that someone must be monitoring his heart rate and vital signs somewhere else. The alarm on the machine was turned off. Dr. O'Malley, the young ER doctor with the casual manner, returned to Ken's room and declared, "Nothing's wrong with you. I think we'll send you home." He explained why it wasn't a heart attack, saying that his blood work showed none of the elevated enzyme levels they look for.

Jennifer was shocked that they would send him home in his current condition, and felt sure that something was terribly wrong. She held her ground, and emphatically told Dr. O'Malley they weren't going anywhere until they had some answers. Dr. O'Malley relented, saying he would repeat the blood tests and they could stay until 3:00. They had given Ken a valium, and he was going back and forth between being lucid and not making sense. Jennifer knew she had to be the advocate and fight for Ken.

July 12, 3:00 P.M.

The next blood test came back with a slightly elevated troponin level, an enzyme they look for with heart attacks. Informing them about the result, Dr. O'Malley said he didn't quite understand it. It might only be a lab error. Yes, he told Jennifer, he had been in touch with the cardiology group that treated Ken, and had spoken to the cardiologist on call. He would order a chest X-ray and additional blood tests to rule out a heart attack once and for all.

Another 30 or 40 minutes later, Dr. O'Malley came in and said, "You need to take your husband home." He assured her that the X-ray appeared normal, telling Jennifer Ken's heart appeared larger than normal, but that was because he was a long-distance runner. The indicators for a heart attack were not there. In fact, his troponin levels had gone back down.

Jennifer felt certain that if she could just force them to keep Ken a little longer, surely the mystery would be solved and they would rush in and fix whatever was wrong with him. She told the doctor they were not leaving; she wanted another blood test to make sure

"There's nothing wrong with him, and you're in our way," the doctor told her.

Again, Jennifer put her foot down and refused to leave. She tried to be as assertive as possible without scaring Ken about his own circumstances. "His hands are ice cold. Something is very wrong!" The frustration and desperation she felt had crept into her voice.

"Fine," he said in a sarcastic manner. "I can humor you and let you stay for one more blood test, and then you've got to go." He didn't order any new tests besides the repeated blood work. No CT scan or MRI. She was appalled by the doctor's attitude, but didn't care if they were only humoring her as long as they let them stay.

The emergency department was busier now, with more activity and more patients. A tanker truck had exploded on I-5, the major north-south interstate. There was a TV outside the room, and Jennifer saw the news footage of the accident on the muted set. Some on the staff were buzzing about it, and she heard them say that the emergency medical technicians were bringing in the truck driver who was involved. No one was paying much attention to Ken as they waited for answers.

July 12, 5:00 P.M.
As they waited for more blood tests, Ken seemed more coherent than

he had all afternoon. He was speaking normally, although Jennifer noticed he was as cold and white as ever.

"I was pretty rattled, wasn't I?" Ken asked her. "I was really confused." His face changed as he said it, and he looked so worried and scared.

"It's alright honey," she reassured him. "They're going to take care of you. You'll be fine." As she said it, she realized she was trying to comfort herself as much as Ken.

"I don't know why I was confused," he said.

In an effort to pass the time, Ken tried to sit up and flip through the pages of a magazine. She asked a nurse for an extra blanket because he was so cold, but the nurse was indifferent and unresponsive, ignoring their request.

"Tell the nurse," Ken turned to his wife. "It's throbbing right here." He tapped the center of his chest. Then he told Jennifer he needed to urinate, and she rang the call button.

When the nurse entered, she was clearly irritated at being summoned. She scowled at Jennifer, and let her know how busy she was, then thrust a urinal at Jennifer telling her she could take care of this. Then she was gone. As Ken urinated, Jennifer was concerned when she noticed his urine was bright orange. A short time later when the nurse returned to empty the urinal, Jennifer held it up and pointed out the orange color. The nurse noted it on Ken's chart. Jennifer again begged for an extra blanket because Ken complained of being so cold, but the nurse left again without acknowledging her request.

July 12, 6:00 P.M.
No one had come to do the final blood test they had been promised. Jennifer rang the call button one more time, and heard a curt reply. "We're busy here. We have codes!"

July 12, 6:15 P.M.
A male nurse came in to take blood. Ken was fumbling with his watch band for some reason, and became upset that he couldn't seem to undo it. The nurse was kind and gentle, and at that point Jennifer was

grateful for someone who treated them with respect and kindness.

"Be thinking about where you want to go to dinner," he told them, an indication that Ken was going to be released shortly. While he began preparing the paperwork for Ken to go home, Jennifer asked him for another blanket. In all this time, no one had brought Ken a blanket. The nurse left and returned quickly with three warm blankets.

Jennifer laid the blankets over Ken and wrapped him tightly, pushing the edges in around his body and feet. His back hurt so, and she turned him gently so she could rub it. She spoke in a soothing voice as she rubbed, telling him it would be alright. About how she would get him home and tuck him into bed, and fix him a home-cooked meal. She kept watching his heart rate, which was still racing. It would go to 200 and even 300 beats per minute. Even now, Jennifer kept imagining if they were patient and waited, someone would see Ken needed help.

July 12, 6:28 P.M.

Ken abruptly began pulling at his IV. "No, no honey. They'll take out the IV," she reminded him. Jennifer put the blankets over his hands to distract him, holding her hands over his under the warm blankets. He was so agitated, and the change had come on quickly.

She took a step back and was about to sit back down in the chair, when Ken's eyes opened wide and he said, "Oh no!" and clutched his sternum.

Jennifer grabbed the call button out from under Ken's body and began screaming for help. No one answered. She left the room and ran to the nurses' station, calling out frantically that her husband needed help, but no one was there. She came back in the room to find Ken seizing with convulsions, and she tried to hold him while begging him not to leave her. Where were they? Why weren't they listening?

The woman in the next bed behind the curtain began yelling, "He's dying! Please help!" Still no one came. Jennifer couldn't find the emergency button—what was it called? Her mind had drawn a complete blank. She couldn't remember the right word to use, as she left again to get help, running down the hall shouting. Then Ken stopped seizing, and fell back on the bed unconscious.

July 12, 6:41 P.M.

On her way out to the hall for the third time, thirteen minutes after Jennifer first called for help, she saw a doctor coming down the hall. It looked like he was with four or five other people. He walked into the room as if nothing had happened. "What's up with him now?" he asked, as if they were a nuisance and he had come to censure them. At first he was looking at Jennifer, not Ken. Then he saw Ken.

The doctor began yelling, "What did he present with? What did he present with?" to the others. "Call a code," he demanded. That was the word Jennifer tried so desperately to remember, but it escaped her during the crisis.

Everything was chaotic. Although Ken had an IV in his left arm, someone was trying to put one in his right. Another person was trying to intubate Ken, but couldn't seem to get the tube in his throat. Two people began CPR. A nurse brought the crash cart to the foot of Ken's bed. She fumbled with the equipment, as she asked a man next to her if he knew how to set it up. Surprised, he asked "Don't you know how to set it up?"

"Can't you people do anything right?" Jennifer cried out, incredulous that their efforts could be so uncoordinated.

There were so many of them in there now. She couldn't help but wonder *where on earth were they before?* All afternoon she had been trying to get someone to look at Ken, to take them seriously and make the effort to find out what was wrong. This is what it took?

A chaplain removed her, guiding her with an arm around her shoulder, and led her to a small, private waiting room nearby.

"It doesn't look good, does it?" Jennifer asked the chaplain.

He gently shook his head and agreed, "No, it doesn't."

July 12, 7:00 P.M.

A few minutes later the doctor came to see Jennifer in the room. They were doing everything they could to save Ken, he told her. Certain that it was a heart attack, he said there was one thing left that they could try but it was risky. As a last resort he could give Ken a clot-busting drug to try and save his life. Willing to try anything, Jennifer told him to go ahead.

July 12, 7:15 P.M.

The doctor returned to tell Jennifer they had lost Ken.

"I'd like to explain to you what happened, to help you feel better," the doctor said quietly.

"Not a word!" she yelled. "Get the hell out of here!" She had never known anger like she felt now. They hadn't listened to her when it mattered, and there was nothing she wanted to hear from them now. Their excuses were pointless.

The phone in the tiny waiting room didn't work she discovered, when she tried to call their son in Seattle. She searched for another phone, and began the grim task of telling the family.

Mark was leaving immediately, he said. His girlfriend, the physician, told him to make sure they did an autopsy as soon as possible, and to get the case notes. Jennifer took her advice. Tracking down their daughter Monique was more challenging, but thankfully Jennifer caught her before she went to a place with no communication. Perhaps the hardest call of all was to Ken's parents. Ken and his father were so close; they were one another's best friends. It would be such a shock. She hadn't even told them he was in the hospital because she didn't want to worry them.

While she waited for Mark, Jennifer spoke with the doctor and staff. The doctor said they would arrange for the autopsy. Jennifer said her son was on his way and she wanted him to see his father.

"But we would have to clean him up, and we're busy," said a doctor. Jennifer said she didn't care, and told them to just do it.

Only the male nurse had been kind, the one who tended to Ken at the end. When Jennifer and Mark went in to see Ken, before they took him away, the nurse came and stood there by the door. By now Jennifer was so accustomed to being treated disrespectfully, she didn't expect anything else.

"Are you here to hurry us up?" she asked the nurse.

"No," he replied. "I'm here to make sure nobody else does either."

Ken Simon's case represents several key points, including misdiagnosis and not listening to the patient and family. In addition, there is a crisis in emergency departments (ED) across the U.S. that comes from being over-taxed and inefficient. In a tragic scenario like the one in Ken's story, a critically ill patient may be camouflaged among the landscape of less seriously ill patients, masking the need for immediate intervention for a life-threatening condition.

Ken had a classic profile of a man presenting with a dissecting aortic aneurysm. An aneurysm, a bulge in a blood vessel, is dangerous because it may burst. The aorta, the main artery leading away from the heart, can develop an aneurysm. Most frequently, aneurysms occur in the abdomen (an abdominal aneurysm), but can also occur in the chest cavity (thoracic aneurysm). This can happen if the wall of the aorta becomes weakened.

In aortic dissection, a tear occurs in the artery wall. These walls consist of three layers: a thin inner layer, a muscular middle layer and a tough outer layer. The tear causes bleeding into and along the aortic wall. In some cases a full rupture can occur, causing bleeding outside the aorta.

Aortic dissection is a life-threatening emergency. When the bulging sac dissects, it causes a person to rapidly lose much of their blood supply as the heart continues to pump blood. If caught early enough, the dissection can be halted through open heart surgery.

This surgery typically involves opening up the dilated portion of the aorta and inserting a synthetic patch. Once the tube in sewn in the aorta, the aneurismal sac is closed around it. Even though the surgery is a high-risk procedure, it is the only alternative in such dire circumstances.

The hospital where Ken was performed open heart surgeries, and had the ability to do an aneurysm repair if the diagnosis had been made quickly. Ken had a significant window of time when they could have attempted to surgically repair the aneurysm. He had the classic presentation of someone with a dissecting aortic aneurysm:

- He was a high risk candidate. He was a male, in his fifties, and had a history of hypertension. In addition, he had an aortic valve insufficiency.
- His chest pain was sudden, mid-sternum, sharp, throbbing. Sometimes the presentation is described as a ripping pain, going into the back, but not in every case.
- He had loss of consciousness, low blood pressure and rapid pulse rate.

Perhaps most importantly, Ken had symptoms that distinguished his aortic dissection from a heart attack. Although some types of heart attacks can affect major nerves and mimic some of these symptoms, they are much more pronounced in an aortic dissection. Specifically, Ken's symptoms showed his blood supply was being diverted, and leaking into his chest:
- Cold, numbness and tingling in the hands and feet (low blood pressure)
- Confusion, tunnel vision, loss of consciousness and inability to speak (lack of blood flow to the brain)
- Orange urine (disrupted blood flow to the kidneys)
- Rapid heart rate and low blood pressure (signs of shock and blood loss)
- Widened area on the chest X-ray (enlarging aorta)

Every one of these symptoms distinguishes Ken's profile from a typical heart attack. From his trip to the hospital to his full cardiac arrest, over six hours passed without an appropriate workup, despite a family member insisting to hospital healthcare professionals that something was seriously wrong.

By Monday, July 14, it was confirmed that Ken suffered a dissecting aortic aneurysm. Mark and Jennifer insisted that the coroner personally call them as soon as he discovered the cause of death. During the autopsy, the coroner interrupted the procedure to phone them, and gave them the results before he had even finished.

As discussed in earlier chapters, misdiagnosis is a central issue in medical errors. However, in addition to the incomplete assessment, and the failure to order appropriate tests to diagnose his problem, the emergency department staff did not heed the warning signs that both Ken and his wife expressed. When she requested her husband's hospital records after his death, Jennifer learned that Ken's x-ray showed an enlarged aorta with a widened area in his chest, another clue that had been ignored.

Ken was mistakenly diagnosed with a panic attack and given valium. Just as the classic presentation of dissecting aortic aneurysm was missed, Ken was far from a classic presentation of someone suffering a panic attack. He was a jet pilot, a man with no current stress in his life, and he had a loving and supportive family. His anxiety was not psychological, but real; he was in shock and felt an impending sense of doom. Indeed, he was dying, and no one helped him.

Although this blatant missed diagnosis and failure to listen cannot be excused, there are two central factors that affect emergency care in the United States, being over-taxed and inefficient. These are crucial issues that lead to medical errors.

According to an Institute of Medicine (IOM) report, there were nearly 114 million visits to U.S. hospital emergency departments in 2003. That's equivalent to one in every three people visiting the ER, and represented an increase from 90.3 million in 1993. These visits range from minor colds to full trauma victims.

As the IOM explains, in addition to critical trauma and life-threatening illnesses, emergency departments have become the safety net for community healthcare services. In that same ten years, the U.S. lost the equivalent of 425 emergency departments, or 198,000 beds, due to closures. These closures are often attributed to the vanishing revenues and quality concerns involved in keeping open an active emergency department.

It is not uncommon in many busy urban, and even rural, emergency departments to see patients lining the hallways on gurneys or in wheelchairs, as the waiting room is packed to overflowing. In some hospitals, emergency personnel occasionally wait up to 30 minutes to offload ambulance patients, a site that was rarely seen even ten years ago. Often, patients that need to be admitted to the hospital wait long hours in the emergency department until an in-patient bed becomes available, leading to further emergency overcrowding.

Ken Simon was lost in the midst of a busy, overloaded emergency department. The truck explosion was dramatic, and may have contributed to the lack of attention. In addition, a meth addict in the ER coded repeatedly and required resuscitation several times, taking the focus away from Ken's deteriorating condition. It's difficult to know what role these other crises played in the physician neglecting to order important tests, or the lack of time and care he received from the staff. None of these distractions excuse the poor care that Ken received, but his scenario demonstrates a problem that is all-too common in hospitals. The issue of emergency department overcrowding and rushed diagnoses places many high-risk patients in peril.

In recent years, two other significant cases related to emergency department problems were in the spotlight. They involved poor screening or delays in treatment that resulted in patient deaths.

In July, 2006, in an Illinois hospital emergency department, 49-year-old Beatrice Vance presented to the ED with symptoms of nausea, shortness of breath and chest pain. The triage nurse assessed Ms. Vance and sent her back to the waiting room. Two hours later, when they finally called her name, she had died form a heart attack and was slumped over in a chair.

In an unusual ruling, a coroner's jury ruled that Ms. Vance' death was a homicide. "Ms. Vance had the classic symptoms of a heart attack," said the coroner of Lake County, Ill. "She should have been in the emergency department much quicker, and received the care that we have in modern medicine." This was the first known case where a hospital was charged with homicide for a delay related to medical care. The Illinois District Attorney's office did not pursue the recommendations of the coroner's jury for homicide charges.

1000%

THE PERCENTAGE INCREASE IN THE NUMBER OF SENTINEL EVENTS RELATED TO DELAYS IN TREATMENT REPORTED TO JOINT COMMISSION BETWEEN 1994 AND 2004.

(Source Joint Commission Sentinel Event Statistics, 2008.)

On May 9 of 2007, in a Los Angeles hospital, Elizabeth Rodriguez, 43, mother of three children, had been seen in the emergency department three times in three days for abdominal pain. She returned to the ED and stood in the lobby, yelling and crying in pain. She wasn't taken back in for an evaluation or examination. While waiting to be seen, Ms. Rodriguez fell to the floor and continued to complain of intense abdominal pain.

She was ignored, even as other people in the waiting room called 9-1-1 to get her emergency help. When a police officer was summoned, he tried to rouse Ms. Rodriguez only to find she had no pulse. Resuscitation efforts failed. The coroner's report said that she died of a perforated and infected large intestine, a treatable ailment that could have been caught sooner.

Due to the federal mandates of EMTALA (Emergency Medical Treatment and Active Labor Act), as discussed in an earlier chapter, moderately to seriously ill patients cannot be turned away from a hospital's emergency department. In addition, the EMTALA regulation has created a culture of fear among hospitals that makes them reluctant to refer even minor illnesses or injuries to other, less costly healthcare services. Intended to help unstable patients and avoid "patient dumping," the law may have contributed to overcrowding and long delays in emergency departments. Using the ED to substitute for a clinic or physician's office has overwhelmed hospital resources and posed dangers for seriously ill patients, as well as contributed to inefficiencies and, no doubt, medical errors.

PROTECT YOURSELF IN TODAY'S HEALTHCARE SYSTEM

Several years after Ken internally bled to death in the emergency department, Jennifer Simon is beginning to come to grips with losing her extraordinary husband. She says that, "Physically, mentally and emotionally, it has cost me beyond words. Every morning waking up without him is almost unbearable."

Jennifer thought long and hard about legal action. She was told she had a good case. But that wouldn't have achieved what she really wanted - changes so this wouldn't happen to another family. She wanted the hospital to learn from their error.

Jennifer asked for a meeting with the hospital administration, to make them hear her out and understand the danger in healthcare professionals ignoring what people tell them. The emergency department doctor and staff hadn't listened to them, or heeded the clear warning signs in Ken's case. By communicating her experience, she felt Ken could go on teaching safety even after his death.

After two meetings with the administration, Jennifer agreed to a small settlement, but she wanted a mark to be made against the physician's record. A hospital official told her that Dr. O'Malley took the event to heart, and really learned from the experience. She was told that he's a different doctor today as a result of what happened.

Jennifer was invited to join a group of patients, family and community members that had formed in 2005. Their focus was and is on patient safety improvements for the healthcare system. Later on, she did a walk-through with the hospital directors to show them safety features they could install that would improve safety, such as code blue buttons in the emergency department examining rooms that would be clearly marked and easily accessible.

The hospital worked with Jennifer and made an educational video about Ken's medical error. It contains compelling interviews with the staff involved in Ken's event, and discusses what went wrong with communication and what can be learned. Jennifer is in the video also. The parent company of the hospital distributed the video to all of its hospitals throughout all its state regions.

A central theme in the video is that healthcare professionals need to listen to patients and their families when they think something is wrong. It goes on to say that communication breakdown is a central issue in medical errors. If a different diagnosis had been made, Ken Simon's life "possibly may have been saved."

Much needs to be done to improve care in emergency departments. People can take strong measures on their own, such as asking for another physician to evaluate them, or even calling their primary physician and asking for help if they feel something is wrong. As discussed in an earlier chapter, a patient or family member can insist to talk to the chief of emergency services, or even the chief of the medical staff, if they feel that something is wrong.

PRESCRIPTION FOR BETTER CARE

The Institute of Medicine (IOM) convened a committee of experts for a period of almost three years, to study the growing crisis in U.S. emergency departments. They consulted other panels of experts, and studied data and trends in emergency department care. Their work resulted in three major conclusions for a future vision of U.S. emergency departments. The IOM recommends:

1. Improved coordination of services and communication. This recommendation discusses the need for an accurate and seamless exchange of information, from pre-hospital through hospital care. Currently, individual areas vary widely in the efficiency of this communication.

2. Regionalization of specific medical services, creating specialized emergency departments modeled after trauma centers, such as stroke or cardiac centers of excellence. Perhaps with a specialized cardiac ED, Ken's condition might have been recognized quickly. Creating specialized centers is complex, and because of geographic limitations may not be easily implemented.

3. Accountability in performance. To build accountability, the IOM committee recommends that the Department of Health and Human Services convene a panel of emergency and trauma experts, who would develop evidence-based indicators of emergency and trauma care performance. Once the data is developed, and appropriately collected and monitored, the results will lead to incentives that reward well-functioning and efficient emergency centers.

The IOM recommendations are broad, sweeping and complex. There are no simple solutions to the growing crisis in emergency care. Most emergency departments that are faced with tough problems have put together performance or operational teams to address and solve issues. Some efforts have helped, such as adding more ED physicians or expanding physical space. Some hospitals have added nurse practitioners, or created clinics within the ED, called fast track or urgent care, to evaluate the more minor illnesses and injuries. While some of these steps have helped to ease overcrowding, some of these solutions are band-aids on a gaping wound.

It's hard to know what might have happened if Ken Simon was diagnosed immediately upon his arrival at the hospital, or even within the first few hours. Perhaps his life might have been saved. Dissecting aortic aneurysms have a high mortality, even with surgical intervention, but he was never given a chance. For a man that dedicated his professional life to improving aviation safety, he should have had that chance.

Like many in-flight crises, dissecting aortic aneurysms are statistically rare, and many physicians go years without seeing a case. Some emergency physicians may only see one or two in a career. An emergency checklist to distinguish heart attack from dissecting aortic aneurysm, much like the emergency checklist Ken wrote, should have been in place for Ken's fairly uncommon diagnosis.

Questionable emergency room care:
- If you feel your emergency department care is inadequate, ask for another emergency room physician to make an evaluation. If no other emergency physician is available, ask to speak to the Chief of Emergency Medical Services or a supervisory committee chair that oversees emergency services. You can also request that the Chief of Staff or Chief Medical Officer be contacted.
- If you feel you are receiving inadequate services in the emergency department, don't hesitate to call your own physician.

Important publications for you to review:
- There are three reports from the Institute of Medicine on the crisis of Emergency Departments in the United States, published by the National Academies Press:
  - *Hospital Based Emergency Care: At the Breaking Point*
  - *Emergency Medical Services: At the Crossroads*
  - *Pediatric Emergency Care: Growing Pains*
- Collectively, the reports describe an overburdened system that is rapidly approaching its limits.
  - Log onto www.iom.edu/emergencycare for more information on the IOM reports
- Many hospitals are moving toward becoming centers for specific specialized services in addition to general medicine and surgery, such as burn units, trauma units, stroke and heart attack centers.
- For more information on aortic aneurysm log onto the Vascular Disease Foundation at: http://www.vdf.org/AAA/

CHAPTER 9

THE PRICE OF DOING

In this chapter
- Learn what preventative measures you and your physician can take before surgery to reduce your risk of hospital acquired infections.
- Find out what factors increase your risk of infection.
- Discover the importance of proper surgical wound care and hygiene.
- Monitor the hygiene practices of hospital healthcare workers while they are providing care.

Why hospital acquired infections are important for you to know about?

An estimated 500,000 surgical site infections occur each year and the mortality rate for such infections stands near 13 percent. In addition, patients acquire infections through catheters, intravenous lines and other medical equipment. The incidence of drug-resistant bacteria continues to grow, making many of these infections increasingly difficult to treat. Healthcare professionals can prevent many infections, but it's up to patients and family members to make sure physicians and nurses take the right steps.

BUSINESS

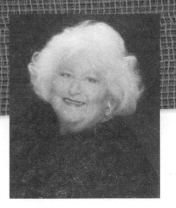

Johanna Daly

The holidays had just passed and it was an early January day, the initial luster of winter had already worn off when Johanna Daly got the idea to take a road trip south, to Disney World in Florida. It would be a girls-only vacation with her two grown daughters, Maureen and Marie, a welcome respite from the cold weather in Brooklyn, New York. They would see the sights and visit some old friends who lived there.

At the age of 63, Johanna was an outgoing, energetic woman who loved to travel. In fact, she and her husband, Danny, were on a mission to visit all fifty states, and now there were just five more to cross off their list. Nothing held them back. Married 43 years, they were at a point where they had the freedom to enjoy their time together. Danny had retired from his work a few years earlier. Their health was good, overall, and although they had lived in the same Brooklyn neighborhood all their lives, they loved adventure.

Danny still thought his wife was the most beautiful woman in the world. Yes, her red hair had turned silvery-white and she had gotten a little older. But she still had the same brilliant blue eyes and a soft welcoming smile, and she was still his Irish rose. In the words of their daughter, Maureen, they were "the corniest and cutest couple."

Both of their parents had come from the same county in Ireland, and their families knew each other when Johanna and Danny were babies. Some years later, Danny, tall and handsome at just 18, spotted his future wife across a crowded dance floor when she was a slender, striking 17-year-old redhead. He made up his mind then and there. After a few dates he asked her to go steady, and told her he was going to marry her someday. Johanna informed him she intended to become a nun. But when she discovered they had their faith and a devotion to the Sacred Heart in common, she figured God might have other plans for her, and Danny didn't have much trouble winning her over. They were very different; she was gregarious and he was an introvert. Their spirituality was the common thread that wove their lives together, and on November 5, 1961, his twenty-second birthday, Daniel Daly married Johanna Sullivan.

On this particular Friday, Danny drove Johanna and Maureen to a nearby mall to shop for vacation clothes. Just looking at the new cruise-wear, hinting at the promise of sun and heat, made them feel closer to the warmth of Florida. After working up an appetite in the stores, Danny offered to buy his girls lunch at a seafood restaurant. All through lunch they talked about what they would do each day on their trip, and how Danny would get along without his beloved "Joanie" to look after him while she was away. After he paid the check, Danny offered to go get the car and bring it around for Maureen and Johanna. Even though it hadn't snowed in over two weeks it was below freezing, and Danny was always chivalrous when it came to the women in his life.

As the women left the restaurant, they made their way down an outside ramp. They hadn't noticed the buildup of ice from a leaking dumpster nearby. Johanna lost her footing on a patch of ice, and her legs went out from under her. She landed on her right shoulder just as her husband arrived with the car.

"Oh, dear Jesus, I can't get up!" she exclaimed, surprised by the swiftness with which it had happened. She felt like the wind was knocked out of her. "Danny, my shoulder is gone."

Danny helped her into the car, while Maureen went inside to report the incident to the restaurant. Her mother yelled behind her, "Tell them they have to take care of it," referring to the glazed ice outside the doorway. It was just like Johanna to be concerned about other people who might get hurt, instead of her own injury.

They first took her to a local hospital in Brooklyn, but Maureen and Danny wanted to make sure she got the best care. The physicians at the hospital determined Johanna had a fractured shoulder, and recommended that she see someone in Manhattan at a specialty hospital. They made an appointment with Dr. Finch, an orthopedic surgeon in the city.

Both Danny and Maureen accompanied Johanna to the appointment. An attractive man with dark eyes and closely cropped hair, Dr. Finch seemed kind and competent, and he exuded the confidence of an experienced surgeon.

As he explained the procedure to repair Johanna's shoulder, she was completely engaged, listening carefully and asking plenty of questions about the surgery. She asked specifics about what would be done and how big the incision would be. She asked about what she could expect during the recovery. Of course her most insistent question was, "When can I go to Florida?" unstoppable as always.

Maureen wondered if this man knew what Johanna meant to their family, how she took care of everyone and how her father lit up when his Joanie walked into a room. Maureen put her arm around her mother, looked directly into Dr. Finch's eyes and said, "You can have my house. You can have my car, my jewelry, my money. None of it means anything without my mother. She is the most precious thing to us, and she has to be alright."

"I can have your house?" Dr. Finch joked as he smiled. He noticed no one else was laughing with him, straightened his face, and quickly said, "Mrs. Daly will be fine."

They scheduled the surgery for Martin Luther King, Jr. Day.

Martin Luther King, Jr. Day, Monday, January 19
On the morning of the surgery the doctor made a change in the plan. He decided he might replace the shoulder instead of repairing it, due to the extent of the damage, and told Johanna and her family. With Maureen and Marie by his side, Danny reluctantly said goodbye to his Joanie and gave her a kiss. Marie, a registered nurse at another healthcare organization, reassured her father that the surgeon and the staff would take good care of her. During the operation the family waited nervously, some of them saying the rosary, until the doctor came out and said it went well. A nurse brought a very relieved Maureen into the recovery room to see her mother.

Wednesday, January 21

Johanna spent two uneventful nights in the hospital before she was due to be released. On the last day, a resident came in to examine and discharge her. Without washing his hands or applying gloves, he ripped off the old dressing to look at the surgical incision, touching and squeezing it as he commented how great it looked. Then he put on a fresh dressing and signed Johanna's discharge papers.

Both Maureen and Johanna silently wondered why the doctor hadn't washed and gloved before treating the wound, but they were both focused on the happy fact that she was going home and didn't say anything. Besides, the surgical site looked like it was healing so well. But when it was time for Johanna to get out of bed and get ready to leave, the two women found the filthy dressing in the hospital bed under the covers. The resident hadn't even bothered to throw it away. They were disgusted, and Johanna told Maureen, "See? This is how much they think of me."

The house where Johanna and Danny lived was a two-family dwelling built in 1906. It was a gracious old house where Maureen had a home downstairs, and Danny and Johanna's home was upstairs on the second floor. Because the stairs would have been difficult for Johanna, Maureen fixed up space for her in her place on the first floor. They planned for her to be there about five days. Danny would sleep on the couch next to Joanie so they wouldn't have to be apart. He was so glad his wife was home, and couldn't bear to be separated. Maureen set up the TV so her mother, who was a news junkie, could watch her favorite cable stations like CNN, or perhaps purchase something on the Home Shopping Network.

For the first four days everything was fine. Johanna was enjoying being there with Maureen, still planning for the Disney World trip. The two women had fun just being together, and Danny was always there for whatever Joanie needed.

At the end of the weekend things turned for the worse in a dramatic way. Johanna was in terrible pain, and became agitated. She cried, saying how badly she hurt, and the pain medication seemed to do nothing. No one slept that night. She didn't have a fever, but the pain continued to intensify. Her first post-operative appointment was scheduled for 8:00 the next morning, and they all tried to hang on, relieved that Johanna would be seen in a few hours.

Monday, January 26

By the time they left for the doctor's appointment at the hospital, Johanna was very weak. Maureen couldn't believe how different her mother was from just a half-day before. This had all happened with no warning. She had to rest on her way to the car. By the time they reached the hospital for her follow-up appointment, she couldn't walk in and they had to get a wheelchair for her. The change was abrupt and worrisome.

In the surgeon's office, the doctor looked at the wound. As he removed the dressing, fluid began to flow from the surgical site, green and foul-smelling, and when he squeezed slightly, even more came oozing out. Maureen panicked when she saw this, and asked the doctor if her mother would lose her arm. He told her to calm down; he would schedule a time later in the day to go in and clean it out. Until then, he would send them down to the urgent care center, since the hospital had no emergency room.

A nurse helped them take Johanna down to the urgent care center in her wheelchair, and they all went into the examining room. A very young doctor entered and introduced himself before removing the dressing. His face looked sober and concerned when he saw Johanna's shoulder. Again, Maureen felt alarmed at the expression on the doctor's face. She told him her mother was having a procedure later to clean out the area, and his reply shocked her when he said Johanna's life was in danger, and her shoulder required an immediate incision and drainage. It was highly infected, he explained, and they couldn't wait until Mrs. Daly was admitted to the hospital because it might be too late. He would have to open it now.

Things moved very quickly from that point. The doctor brought in a tray of instruments and asked Danny and Maureen to leave, but Maureen insisted on staying by her mother's side. Danny went back to the waiting area, as the doctor prepared to open the wound. Johanna was already in such pain. Maureen asked the doctor if he was going to give her something before the procedure. He apologized, but said he didn't have any anesthetic readily available there; Maureen would have to help hold her mother still while he drained the infection. Events were moving so quickly. Maureen couldn't believe the doctor was going to do this here, and with no anesthetic.

Johanna's screams could be heard in the waiting area, and Danny went pale at the sound. Back in the examining room, Maureen used her entire body to help hold down her mother, who was writhing on the table. The doctor cut open the incision and more of the disgusting, foul discharge poured out of the surgical wound. He apologized for the pain he had to inflict. Johanna's concern was for Maureen, and she begged her daughter to leave because she didn't want her to have to see and smell the horrible mess. But Maureen assured her she wasn't going anywhere, and continued to hold her. Despite the doctor's efforts to contain the fluid to a basin, it seemed to go everywhere, leaking all over Johanna's clothing and any nearby surfaces in the room. Maureen noticed there was over a pint of fluid in the basin when the doctor finished.

After Johanna was admitted to the hospital and given IV antibiotics, another surgery followed that evening. They cleaned out the wound more completely, and the doctor told Danny and Maureen it went well and she would be fine. It was an encouraging sign that Johanna was talking in the recovery room late that night.

Tuesday, January 27

Danny sent Maureen home to freshen up and get some rest. The staff was going to move Johanna into a hospital room and he could stay with her. Around mid-morning, as they wheeled her through the hallway to her room, Johanna suddenly grabbed Danny's arm and pulled hard. Between gasps of air she managed to say, "I can't breathe! Get me help."

A respiratory therapist happened to be there in the same hallway, and seeing Johanna's distress he ran to her gurney. He saw that she couldn't breathe and noticed her pallor, and insisted they rush her to the intensive care unit immediately. She was burning with fever, so hot that when Danny drew close he could feel the heat rising off of her body. When she arrived in the ICU, the nurse discovered her temperature was 106 degrees. Danny wondered how his wife's condition could have deteriorated this far in just hours. Alone and anxious, Danny phoned the family and told them to come back to the hospital.

By the time Maureen and Marie arrived, Johanna had been placed on a ventilator and was in critical condition. When they saw the state their mother was in, the two girls called their Aunt Kathleen and told her she needed to come right away if she wanted to see her sister alive. The doctor said she was suffering from a major infection. It had traveled from the surgical site in her shoulder through her bloodstream, and had affected her breathing. The doctors were racing against time, using blood tests and cultures from the wound in an effort to find out what specific organism was making her sick. Only then would they have a clearer idea about which drugs would knock it out.

They discovered Joanna was a victim of multi-organism sepsis, and was infected by MRSA, Klebsiella and Pseudomonas, all of them resistant to multiple antibiotics. She had acquired the infections while in the hospital, the very place where she should have been safe.

Valentine's Day, February 14
In the weeks that followed, Danny firmly believed his Joanie would get well and come home soon. He couldn't afford to think otherwise; she was the center of his life. Although she was still on a ventilator in the ICU attached to multiple IV lines and catheters, she was alert and aware. Doctors continued to treat her with antibiotics for the infection and medication for her blood sugar.

By the middle of February Johanna still was unable to move anything but her head, although she kept trying. Because they were corny, hopeless romantics, Valentine's Day had always been special to Danny and Johanna. This year was no exception. He brought her a beautiful Valentine and balloons, and while she seemed pleased by it, she also seemed to get agitated when she looked at it. Maureen was there and asked her mother what was wrong. Although she couldn't talk because of the ventilator and couldn't motion with her hand, Johanna used her head to motion toward the tokens of love that Danny had brought. What was she trying to tell them? Maureen found herself playing a combination of 20 questions and charades to get to the bottom of the mystery. Johanna wanted her daughter to buy Danny a Valentine's card and present it to him on her behalf.

Maureen left in search of something for her mother to give her dad and returned a short time later. She could tell how badly Johanna wanted to sign the card. Carefully, Maureen lifted her mother's limp hand and placed the pen in it, then enfolded it in her own strong hand and guided the pen across the card. They knew then that she understood everything, and somehow that made the situation even harder. Her mind was trapped in a body that no longer responded or worked.

Saturday, February 28

The doctors had been trying to wean Johanna off the ventilator, and by the end of February they took her off completely. Able to talk now for the first time in weeks, she spoke like a stroke victim, with labored speech that was slow and slurred. The plan was to move Johanna to a rehabilitation facility on March 1, where she could receive ongoing therapy and care.

On this day the family was all together in Johanna's room, talking about how this date had been Johanna's mother's birthday. They reminisced about Nana and the old days in Brooklyn, the people and places that were part of the family history they all shared. Danny stayed on after Maureen and the others went home. Maureen had barely set foot in her house when the phone rang.

"Mommy just coded," her father said on the other end of the line. His voice was a mixture of quiet panic and bewilderment.

When Maureen got back to the hospital she learned they were able to resuscitate her mother, and now they were taking her to surgery to perform a permanent tracheostomy so she could breathe. They also intended to put in a feeding tube. The sepsis had ravaged Johanna's organs, and compromised her ability to breathe and swallow, as well as move her extremities. She wasn't responding well to the antibiotics prescribed by the infection specialist. On top of everything else she had developed Clostridium difficile, a spore forming bacteria in the intestines, from the extended use of high-dose antibiotics. It produces toxins in the body.

Thursday, March 4

Once again, Johanna was back in the ICU recovering from surgery, and would remain there for several weeks. Her family was frustrated by the way she was treated by the doctors and staff. Because she couldn't move or speak, they acted as if she couldn't understand anything. But nothing could have been further from the truth.

Johanna still watched television, and her family would sometimes turn on the TV in her room, tuning it to the cable news stations she always enjoyed before. They knew she was following what went on, even if it wasn't immediately apparent to others at the hospital. She was able to say a word here and there with great difficulty, and Maureen had become an expert at interpreting her mother's limited vocabulary.

That morning Johanna shifted her head uneasily in an effort to motion toward the TV. Maureen leaned closer to hear the word her mother was trying to form. Leaning in and watching Johanna's lips, she clearly heard her say "Martha." Danny and Maureen couldn't help smiling when they realized she was referring to Martha Stewart. She somehow remembered that this was the day the "Domestic Diva" would be sentenced, and she wanted to know what happened. Danny turned on the news for her and tried to take some comfort from the fact that his Joanie was as sharp as ever.

Although the doctors said they were "using everything in their arsenal," the infections were persistent. One infection would be under control and another would begin to flourish. Because they were treating four or five different varieties, getting rid of them completely was an elusive goal.

Sunday, March 14

It was Johanna's 64th birthday. Danny was determined to celebrate, despite the fact that she was still in the ICU. Armed with everything he needed for a party—cake, presents, balloons—he showed up at the hospital with the family. His devotion to his wife never wavered. He still had faith they would make her better, and he showed up with his coffee each morning at the same time to sit with her and visit. Joanie would light up when he came in, and Danny would tell her, "That smile is my whole world."

The family had insisted that specialists evaluate Johanna for a stroke while she was there. With her apparent paralysis and difficulty speaking, it seemed like a distinct possibility. After extensive testing, they found no evidence of stroke. Instead, the diagnosis was critical illness neuropathy, a complication of the sepsis. In other words, the infection had permanently damaged her nervous system.

The infection specialist said that in her weakened condition, Johanna was in danger of the infections coming back. She was no longer on a ventilator, and the doctors had applied a tracheostomy collar to hold her breathing tube firmly in place. The doctors wanted to discharge her to a sub-acute hospital for rehabilitation. But the Daly family held their ground, and insisted she stay in acute care rehabilitation. There she was able to receive physical therapy, speech therapy and care for her tracheostomy.

Easter Sunday, April 11

So many holidays had passed in the hospital. For a woman who always made the most of those times, who had up to five Christmas trees in the house each December and even dressed up the dogs in holiday finery, it seemed particularly cruel to be missing one celebration after another.

That year Marie's birthday happened to fall on Easter Sunday, making it twice as special. As always, Johanna was concerned about others, and in her own way let Maureen and Danny know they should do something special for Marie. But for Marie, the best gift was simply having her mother say "Happy Birthday" to her, even if the words no longer came out easily.

Nearly 30 days after Johanna went into acute care rehabilitation, the doctors and staff arranged a conference with the family to discuss her care. The doctors told Danny and his daughters that Johanna's prognosis for further improvement was very poor, and there was nothing more they could do for her there. Danny collapsed sobbing when they said she had to leave. There was now a small, painful crack in his protective armor of hope.

They found a place for her at a rehabilitation hospital on Staten Island, and prepared to move her there. It would do until they could arrange to bring her home. Maureen and Marie understood what the new reality was, and they would spend the next month getting the house ready for their mother's continuing and permanent needs. But for his part, Danny still hoped for a miracle.

Maureen lodged a complaint with the hospital administration in writing, and demanded to meet with them. Before Johanna left the hospital, Maureen sat down with the hospital vice president and the risk manager; the hospital CEO would not see her. She wanted answers, an explanation for how a routine surgery on a healthy woman resulted in such a devastating outcome. Her mother had come in there as a strong, vibrant 63-year-old woman and had left a quadriplegic, unable to speak, breathe or eat normally. And it was all the result of infections she acquired in the hospital.

The risk manager told her that hospital infections were part of "the cost of doing business." They both let her know that nothing short of a court order would cause them to give her additional information. Maureen was appalled by their lack of concern, and furious that the hospital took no responsibility for what had happened to her mother. They didn't even seem surprised that it had happened, or for that matter, sorry.

Maureen asked them to come and see Johanna before she left for the rehabilitation facility. On the morning Johanna was leaving the hospital, the chief administrator refused to come and see Johanna and the family, communicating with them through an impersonal letter.

Both daughters worked tirelessly all through the month of May, transforming Maureen's downstairs home into a suitable place for their mother. They got new furniture that would be comfortable for Johanna, and painted a beautiful mural of an outdoor scene on one wall, so she could feel like she had a window on the world. It was going to be much more difficult for her to get outside now, and bringing the outdoors inside might keep her from feeling cooped up. Accents of green and purple, Johanna's favorite colors, were everywhere. If they kept up at this pace, it would be ready for her scheduled homecoming on May 26.

One day in early May when Maureen was visiting her mother, she found it particularly difficult to squelch the pain of seeing her there, so completely altered and alone. All the feelings she'd been tamping down inside of her came welling up unexpectedly. Maureen began to cry, and placing her hands on her mother's cheeks she said, "My heart is broken for you."

Johanna looked deeply into Maureen's eyes, and as clearly as she had said anything in months, she replied, "And mine is broken for you."

Maureen knew in that moment that they would lose her.

May 9, Mother's Day
Danny and the girls came out to the rehabilitation hospital to spend the day with Johanna. Never without a gift for her on special occasions, Danny brought delicate snowmen made of fine china to add to her collection. Joanie loved snowmen. He was still in love and so eager to please. Maureen and Marie brought an entire menagerie of their mother's pets to visit, three cats and a dog. She had missed them for so long.

Saturday, May 15
The following weekend, Danny was visiting there when his wife seemed distressed. He could tell she was having trouble breathing once again and got the nurse. They called 9-1-1 as they worked to assist her breathing, and Johanna left the rehabilitation facility in an ambulance bound for a university hospital on Staten Island. She was diagnosed with pneumonia, and would remain there for several days while they fought the infection in her lungs.

During the next week it seemed that Johanna had stabilized and improved. The new décor at the house was almost ready for her, and she was expected to come home on May 26. Danny just wanted her home.

Friday, May 21
When Maureen came to visit, her mother appeared to be very sleepy. She couldn't wake her up or get a reaction. At last she seemed to

come to life, and after a short stay Maureen said goodbye, reminding Johanna that they were getting everything ready for her return. "I'll see you Sunday," she told her as she left.

Saturday, May 22

By morning Johanna was more alert. A nurse had combed her hair and placed a yellow ribbon in it, and when Danny came in and saw her, he almost forgot for a moment that she wasn't the same Joanie. They spent much of the day alone together, just the two of them like old times. That rarely happened anymore, as there was little privacy in hospitals and rehab centers. He talked to her about plans for more trips, about visiting the final five states they had yet to see. "Joanie, you look so beautiful," he told her again and again, and she smiled for him each time. Danny held her hand and said how much he loved her. But by evening she had a fever, and he thought briefly about what the infectious disease specialist had said weeks before about her susceptibility to more infections. It was time for him to go home and let her rest.

Sunday, May 23

Maureen was acutely aware that she had just three days before Johanna would be home, and there was still work to do. She started early so she would have time to go visit like she had promised her mother. The phone rang, and her father was on the other end. "Maureen, Mommy died," he said through his tears, and the sound of loneliness in his voice was more than she could bear. Danny had arrived to see his Joanie bright and early that morning, coming straight from 7:15 Mass, and she was gone.

PAYING THE PRICE

In little more than four months, Johanna Daly regressed from a fully-functioning wife and homemaker to an invalid to deceased. The speed and nature of her rapid descent left her family reeling.

Maureen Daly attempted to get answers from the CEO and the risk manager at the specialty hospital in Manhattan. Throughout and after Johanna's hospitalizations, Maureen wrote multiple letters and met with hospital administrators. When Johanna was in the rehabilitation hospital, the CEO sent Maureen a letter that communicated an attitude of carelessness and arrogance, with multiple misspellings including the spelling of Johanna's name. Although the hospital risk manager told Maureen that infections occur everyday in every hospital and are simply the price of doing business, for the Daly family, this price was too high.

Surgical site infections, those involving an incision after surgery, are far too common. According to the Centers for Disease Control (CDC), there are approximately 500,000 surgical site infections each year in U.S. hospitals. With the mortality rate for patients as high as 13 percent and a price tag of more than a billion dollars each year, surgical site infections (SSI) are a major health concern. Additionally, infection rates of up to 11 percent are reported for certain types of operations. Each infection is estimated to increase a hospital stay by an average of seven days, and can add thousands and tens of thousands of dollars in charges.

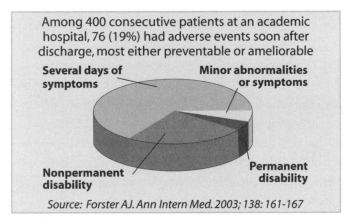

Among 400 consecutive patients at an academic hospital, 76 (19%) had adverse events soon after discharge, most either preventable or ameliorable

Several days of symptoms

Minor abnormalities or symptoms

Nonpermanent disability

Permanent disability

Source: Forster AJ. Ann Intern Med. 2003; 138: 161-167

Johanna Daly developed a surgical site infection that may have been preventable. The problem of more drug-resistant microbes, especially methicillin-resistant S. aureus (MRSA), continues to grow and plague healthcare organizations throughout the world. The prevalence of these and other pathogens, such as gram negative Pseudomonas, Klebsiella, vancomycin-resistant enterococci (VRE) and other resistant organisms is a threat within hospitals. These organisms often affect people with weakened immune systems, but healthy people are not exempt from developing a serious infection either. Some infections are now resistant to all types of antibiotics.

Any of these organisms, alone or in combination, have the

potential to cause sepsis, which can lead to the destruction of multiple organs in the body. Johanna Daly suffered from massive complications in her heart, lungs and kidneys, ultimately leading to a fatal bout with pneumonia. Factors that contribute to these infections can occur directly before, during or after an operation. The most important factors in the prevention of surgical site infections are excellent hygiene and surgical practices.

REDUCING HOSPITAL ACQUIRED INFECTIONS

Surgical Site Infections are so prevalent within hospitals that the CDC is working aggressively with healthcare organizations, researchers and hospital infection control programs to prevent and reduce infections. The CDC's goal is to reduce hospital infections by 50 percent over the next five years.

The CDC asks for public comment on many of their projects. In many states, infections acquired in the hospital must be publicly reported so consumers will have access to that information. In other states the infection rate is reported to authorities, but kept confidential and not available to the general public. This is done to protect hospitals in effort to ensure greater compliance in reporting. It is wise to check the laws and practices governing infection reporting in your state. With approximately one out of ten patients affected by hospital acquired infections, leaders in the healthcare community who commit resources, time and technology to this problem are certain to see returns on their investment.

The consumer should be on the alert for the risk for developing a Surgical Site Infection during a hospital stay, as well as ways to prevent such complications. Healthcare professionals and patients can partner to reduce the chance for infection.

- Use excellent hand hygiene.
- Be informed about pre-surgery antibiotics and the timing for their administration.
- Understand the importance and use of preventative (prophylactic) antibiotics right after surgery.
- Take good care of any catheters, intravenous lines or drainage

tubes, and make sure they are removed as soon as possible when no longer necessary. Work with your doctor on having this done.
• Ask about proper care for all incisions, and ask about accepted guidelines for the removal of staples, stitches and sterile strips.

Maureen is now actively involved with an organization dedicated to reducing hospital infections, Reduce Infection Deaths (RID). RID was founded to:
• Motivate hospitals to make infection prevention a top priority, showing them the benefits and financial savings.
• Provide patients with information on how to protect themselves.
• Educate future doctors and nurses on the precautions needed to stop bacteria from spreading from patient to patient.

PROTECT YOURSELF IN TODAY'S HEALTHCARE SYSTEM

The Centers for Disease Control (CDC) recommends the use of preventative, or prophylactic, antibiotics prior to specific types of surgery. The CDC has compiled evidence from multiple scientific research sources, recommending the administration of a pre-operative antibiotic within one hour of the time a patient undergoes surgery. This is known to prevent infections. Antibiotics administered earlier or later than this time frame have proven not to be as effective as those given within the hour of when surgery begins. In addition, the CDC recommends that prophylactic antibiotics be given for only 24 hours after surgery for most types of procedures.

The prolonged use of antibiotics for routine procedures has not proven effective, and may even be dangerous, increasing the likelihood of antibiotic-resistant infections such as Clostridium difficile (C. diff.), which can cause severe illness. It's important to have a frank discussion with the surgeon performing the procedure prior to the surgery, to review the antibiotic regimen.

Hospitals that treat Medicare patients are required to publicly report their use of prophylactic antibiotics for the following types of procedures: colon, heart, vascular, hip, knee and gynecology. These rates are listed on the CMS website at: http://www.hospitalcompare .hhs.gov/

The surgical technique utilized is a critical factor in surgical site infection prevention. Four critical preventative areas exist: skin preparation, hair removal, operating room practices and post-operative wound care. Skin has natural bacteria, including organisms like Staphylococcus aureus. Although all surgeries require some type of skin preparation to remove this surface bacteria, several studies have shown that a preoperative wash containing chlorhexidine decreases the bacterial count on the skin by as much as 80 to 90 percent.

Another key preventative factor that cannot be over emphasized is the method used for hair removal prior to surgery. It is now well established that shaving damages skin, and increases the growth of bacteria. When hair needs to be removed, clipping the hair close to the surface without damaging the skin is the preferred method for skin preparation. Prior to having any surgery, it is important to question and stop anyone who attempts to prepare the skin by using any kind of razor.

The cause of Johanna's surgical site infection was never released to the Daly family by the hospital. An internal review was completed, and Maureen reported the infection to the Joint Commission. Surgical site infections are considered significant events, and warrant a serious investigation. Many states, such as Pennsylvania, Indiana and California, now require hospitals to report these infections, especially if they result in patient harm. Maureen made a report to the New York Department of Health Services (DHS) and to the Joint Commission, although neither organization provided her details about the results or cause related to her mother's death.

It is likely that the Joint Commission conducted a thorough review and evaluation of operating room practices at the hospital, including instrument sterilization, appropriate aseptic technique and other processes. A breech in any of these practices could lead to a surgical site infection.

Finally, but just as important, is the appropriate management of an incision after surgery. This includes the proper use of surgical dressings and scrupulous hand hygiene. Maureen's observation of the resident removing Johanna's surgical dressing without washing his hands was significant. No one will know for sure if that encounter introduced an antibiotic-resistant organism to Johanna's incision, but it most certainly presented an opportunity for infection.

The development of infections varies widely from hospital to hospital, surgeon to surgeon, type of procedure and the risk factors of patients. All facilities have some incidence of infection. However, certain practices may help reduce the occurrence of Surgical Site Infections. Here are a few critical safeguards to consider before having surgery:

- Control blood glucose before, during and after surgery.
- Stop all tobacco use 30 days before surgery.
- Improve nutritional status prior to a surgical procedure.
- Shower or bathe the night before or morning of the operation using chlorhexidine soap, which can be purchased at any drugstore or pharmacy.
- Taper or discontinue systemic steroid use before elective surgery (talk to your doctor if you are on a steroidal medication).
- Talk to your surgeon about the antibiotics he/she will use prior to and post-surgery.
- Do not remove hair from the surgical site unless necessary. If hair is removed, make sure it is done immediately before surgery, preferably with electric clippers. Question anyone if they attempt to use a razor for hair removal (talk to your healthcare team about this).
- Keep you preoperative stay in the hospital as short as possible.
- Work with your surgeon to keep your hospitalization after surgery as brief as possible.
- Ask all healthcare workers to wash their hands or use hand gel before changing dressings, caring for you or touching your incision.

Protecting yourself against hospital acquired infections following surgery:

- Meet with your surgeon prior to surgery. Ask what antibiotic you need and what time you need it. Make sure your doctor prints out the drug name and time it should be administered. Take this paper with you to the hospital to show the anesthesiologist and each of the nurses preparing you for surgery.
- If you have an incision from a procedure or surgery, strictly follow the instructions you have been given.
- Ask clinicians and healthcare workers caring for you to wash their hands or use hand gel any time they have direct contact with you.
- If you are in the hospital, wash your hands frequently and thoroughly. If you are unable to get out of bed, ask a nurse or aide for antiseptic hand sanitizer.
- When you wash your hands, sing the song *Yankee Doodle Dandy*. This is great for children as well. Otherwise, wash your hands briskly for 15 to 30 seconds.
- If you have had a surgical site infection you can report this to The Joint Commission and to your state Department of Health Services. To contact Joint Commission log onto: http://www. jointcommission.org/AboutUs/ContactUs/

For more information on the Centers for Disease Control and their work on the reduction of infections log on to: www.CDC.gov/ drugresistance

To learn more about RID, log onto http://www.hospitalinfection.org

CHAPTER 10

WRONG TURN

In this chapter
- Learn how to do your part to reduce your chances for wrong-site/wrong-side surgery.
- Learn what factors increase your risk for such mishaps.
- Find out why you should carefully read all hospital paperwork before signing it.
- Discover the importance of verifying and marking the surgical site.
- Learn about the Universal Protocol that all hospitals should use in the operating room and procedure areas.

Why having the right type of surgery on the correct body part is crucial for you to know?
Surgical procedures on the wrong part of the body are more common than the public may realize; but accurate statistics are not available. National estimates range from several hundred to several thousand wrong site/wrong side surgeries each year. In one survey of physicians, 21 percent admitted to performing surgery on the wrong body part. Ultimately, it is up to the patient and family members to ensure physicians and nurses have the correct information when they are preparing the patient for surgery.

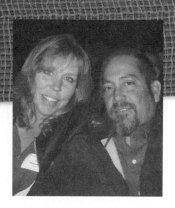

Benjamin and Monica Houghton

It had been a warm June day when Benjamin Houghton awoke in the recovery room to find three doctors at his bedside. The sober looks on their faces told him something was very wrong. As one of them started to speak, Benjamin learned why they were there surrounding his bed. For a moment he wasn't quite sure he heard the doctor correctly. Maybe he was still feeling the effects from the anesthesia they gave him during his surgery.

"This is a joke, right?" he asked the doctors, waiting for one of them to say it was some kind of sick prank.

"No, I'm afraid this is no joke," another doctor replied. "There was a mix-up. We accidentally removed the wrong testicle."

"Get my wife. Get Monica" Benjamin said. Monica will sort this all out, he thought. She'll figure out what's going on. It can't possibly be as drastic as what they're saying. Things like this just don't happen in real life.

Monica was his rock. They met years before when Benjamin was diagnosed with testicular cancer the first time. He had been in the military then, an MP in the Air Force. At 29 years old, he was divorced with two young children. The doctors had told him he had cancer, and then had flown him to Andrews Air Force Base for his initial care. There was no surgery that time, only the dreaded treatments at a Veterans Administration hospital in Sepulveda. Ben's father drove him to and from the hospital for his treatments. But it was Monica who really got him through the ordeal. In fact, it was actually the children who brought them together in the beginning.

He was undergoing chemotherapy, and needed a monitor for his son and daughter, aged three and five. Monica had a young four-year-old daughter as well. Their friendship deepened, and by the time he was in remission and feeling well a year later, they were in love and decided to marry. That was 15 years ago.

Now they made their home in Frazier Park and had two more children, a 13-year-old son and a daughter who was eight. The older kids were out of the house for the most part, his two living in San Bernardino, and her daughter away at college, and Monica worked for a cruise line in Valencia. Although Ben continued to experience some pain in the affected testicle over the years, blood tests showed that the cancer was still in remission and had not spread. He felt very lucky.

Ben experienced renewed concern about the cancer in November 2005, when he was hospitalized with diabetes. The pain had increased in his atrophied testicle, where the cancer had been before, and he had developed abdominal pain. They performed an ultrasound while he was in the V.A. hospital and felt that for safety they should remove the testicle in case the cancer was back. They made a decision to operate. Ben was told he would need to have the affected testicle removed this time, a procedure called an orchiectomy. Since their family was complete, Ben decided to have a vasectomy at the same time.

Doctors at a V.A. Medical Center in Southern California area attempted to do the surgery in February of 2006, but there were complications with the anesthesia and intubation. It was frightening for Monica when a doctor pulled her into the hallway to explain what had gone wrong. They had to suspend Ben's surgery and reschedule it for a later date.

When Ben and Monica arrived for surgery the next time, the procedure was cancelled at the last minute. Each time he had to wait, Ben became more anxious. It was difficult to mentally prepare for something like that, only to have it postponed and face it all over again.

Now it was June 14. It seemed that this time things would go smoothly. Ben and Monica made the long drive from their home in Frazier Park to another Veteran's hospital, grateful it was early and the worst of the traffic hadn't yet started. They arrived at the V.A. hospital campus, parking in a lot near the block looking building where he would spend the night. As much as he dreaded the surgery, Ben looked forward to the absence of pain, the pain he had learned to tolerate these past months. The discomfort even made it difficult to walk normally, causing him to limp.

In the prep room Dr. Singer, the surgeon and fifth-year surgical resident, handed Ben some routine paperwork to sign. Ben took the clipboard from the doctor, but realized he couldn't see what the paperwork said.

"I don't have my reading glasses," Ben told him.

The surgeon assured Ben it was the same consent form with the same information that he had signed the last time he was there, when his surgery was postponed. They had previously discussed everything that was included. Ben hesitated, but figured that Dr. Singer knew what he was talking about. A nurse handed him a pen and he signed on the bottom of the form.

After being wheeled into the operating room, Ben was asked by a masked nurse to point out the site of the operation. He pointed to his left testicle, but no one marked the area. That was the last thing Ben remembered before the anesthesiologist asked him to count backward, as he administered a drug into Ben's IV line that would send him off to sleep.

Now that he was awake and fully aware, Ben's very real nightmare had begun. Monica entered the recovery room escorted by a nurse. Her long, wavy blonde hair looked disheveled, like she had been napping in the waiting room during his surgery. She looked as confused as he felt. Her eyes were wide with surprise under a furrowed brow.

The three doctors again began to explain that there had been "a mistake."

"We accidentally removed the right testicle and . . ." one of them said.

Monica struggled to understand. "But there was nothing wrong with the right one," she interrupted before the doctor could go any further.

"There was a mix-up with the consent. The vasectomy and orchiectomy were switched. We did the opposite. The right testicle was removed instead of the left."

"Aren't you supposed to mark the area?" Monica couldn't believe this.

The doctors continued with their explanation, apologizing for the confusion and assuring them the hospital would provide all the medical services he would need in the future.

"What am I supposed to do now?" Ben asked the surgeons. This was surreal; it couldn't be happening.

A mistake! As the reality of the wrong-side surgery began to sink in, it became clear what this error meant for Ben; he was castrated. His one healthy, functioning testicle had been removed, and the cancerous, atrophied one had been left behind. *How the hell could this happen*, he thought.

He had trusted the doctors. Ben and Monica had confidence in the V.A. system. They were supposed to be national leaders in patient safety, using electronic medical records and the latest technology to prevent medical errors. The V.A. had received the national Gold Seal award from the national inspectors.

As their shock subsided, their first concern was finding out what Ben would need to recover, and getting him the follow-up care he would require in the wake of such a devastating loss. Monica turned her attention to supporting Ben and researching his condition, gathering any information she could lay her hands on. The Internet was an invaluable resource in learning about castration and its treatment.

Because Ben would no longer produce natural testosterone, he would need to take supplemental testosterone for the rest of his life. These hormone replacements were not without their own negative side effects. Testosterone replacements, they learned, carry the risk of stimulating both benign and malignant prostate tumor growth. In addition, they can reduce HDL cholesterol levels, the "good" cholesterol, and are associated with an increased risk of coronary artery disease.

But without the testosterone supplements, Ben discovered he was at greater risk for osteoporosis and broken bones. Without testosterone his sexual desire and ability to perform would greatly diminish or disappear entirely. He might suffer from significant depression and mood swings. It was like a male menopause, but far worse because it was not a natural process. The absence of testosterone could cause other health complications including fatigue, memory loss, weight gain and loss of muscle strength.

The only positive thing Ben read about castration was that it stopped male-pattern baldness. Although, he joked, it was too late for him because he already had a receding hairline. Monica was amazed that he could find something to laugh about. Ultimately, Ben realized his only alternative would be to take the hormone supplements and watch carefully for their side effects.

None of the available delivery systems were perfect for taking the testosterone supplements. Ben found that the patches and gels blistered and irritated his skin. While he could use injections, they were difficult to administer and painful.

Ben's recovery was slow and uneven. Monica and the kids recognized that he had good days and bad days. Because of the injury he suffered, Ben was forced to file for disability while Monica continued to work for the cruise line. His energy ebbed, and his mood and attitude fluctuated. It became more difficult for Ben to control his temper and he lacked patience. He became more introverted, not interacting with the family as much as he had before. Ben and Monica's relationship began to change under the strain. He feared losing his marriage, although Monica tried to be supportive and reassuring.

To add to his physical problems, Ben still had significant pain in the existing diseased testicle. At times, the pain was so severe it caused him to limp. He developed an awkward gait to compensate for the discomfort.

As Ben and Monica investigated what happened, their anger grew over what they discovered about the wrong-side surgery. It was clear from the beginning of the pre-surgical phase what procedures were to be done, and on what side. Because Ben had the cancer in his left testicle since 1989, he had extensive records at the V.A. indicating the cancer treatment and atrophy. All his medical records and tests were contained at the Southern California V.A. hospital, so there should have been no mistake about which side of the body required surgery.

Monica researched wrong-side surgery, and realized there should have been a process in place to mark the correct side that was to be operated on. No one did this. When Monica asked about why this hadn't been done, she was told Ben's surgical area was "private," and for this reason the pre-surgical team avoided marking or discussing the area. This was both frightening and astounding, and further infuriated Ben and Monica. These were healthcare professionals, for goodness' sake. Didn't they operate on breasts, pelvic organs and other so-called "private parts" every day?

They found out there were many ways the team could have marked the site to indicate the correct side, such as marking above the affected testicle or marking the leg on the correct side. But these measures were not taken either. The more they learned the more they realized that they needed to seek legal action.

Ben and Monica found a uniquely qualified attorney to represent them, one who was a physician as well as a lawyer, Susan Friery, MD from the law firm of Kreindler & Kreindler. They wanted someone to protect their rights so they could accomplish two goals; they wanted to assure Ben's medical care would be covered at a facility of their choice, and they wished to help prevent this type of error from occurring to anyone else. They filed a claim against the V.A. hospital, to cover the costs of Ben's future healthcare outside the Department of Veterans Affairs system. Their attorney also helped them contact the media to tell their story, believing this was one way they could help others to avoid the same kind of terrible mistake.

As required by V.A. policy for errors in such cases, the hospital arranged a meeting in which they must sit with the patient and family, and formally apologize to them for what had happened. Along with the Houghton's, those present included the senior attending urologist and the chief of staff for the V.A. system. The doctor who was personally responsible for the mistake was absent.

The hospital's apology was perfunctory, lasting only 30 seconds, and lacked any genuine compassion or feeling. No questions were allowed, and Ben was told he really should have the other testicle removed—at a V.A. hospital, of course. After what had happened, Ben was more than reluctant to place his care in their hands. Instead of the meeting becoming a starting point for healing and understanding, it was a meaningless exercise. Ben and Monica left feeling worse than when they came.

For its part, the hospital has made a switch to electronic consent forms now, so that information from the patient's records is automatically transferred to the consent forms without the risk of a transcription error. The surgeon must now review the information on the consent form, match it against the patient's chart, and consult the patient for agreement.

Ben and Monica continue to live with Ben's side effects and complications every day. Their lives are forever changed following this preventable medical error and although a settlement was reached, the process was cold and calculated and lacked the true compassion a patient might expect under such circumstances. Ben's trust in the healthcare system has been permanently jaded, yet he has many medical conditions that require frequent care. However, he is now extremely cautious and still fears for those who are not alert to all the medical errors that are prevalent in today's U.S. health systems.

There were multiple high-risk points in the sequence of events that led to Benjamin Houghton's wrong-side surgery:

- A dual procedure involving both testicles was being performed, increasing the risk of wrong-site surgery. This should have signaled the need to verify the surgical sides with greater intensity.
- Ben's consent information was carried over several times when his surgery was postponed. The consent was never re-verified with the patient.
- The completion of the consent form was incorrect; Ben did not have his glasses, the consent should have been read to him orally in the presence of his wife, and Ben made the assumption that the information was correct. Assumptions should never be made when dealing with consent forms.
- Extra verification should have occurred at this point, comparing his diagnostic tests with the correct sides to be operated on. This didn't occur.
- The immediate Universal Protocol done before surgery was incomplete and incorrect. Ben pointed to the correct side (left), but nothing was marked. Despite him pointing to the correct side, they continued to follow the wrong information on the consent form.
- The medical records showed that a time-out was performed, but it's unclear whether the surgical team consulted any document besides the erroneous consent form.

The consent form prepared on the day of surgery stated that the right testicle was to be removed, and a left-side vasectomy performed. It should have stated the opposite. The records did not say who prepared the consent

16%

THE PERCENTAGE OF SURVEYED PHYSICIANS WHO SAID THEY HAD ACCIDENTLY PREPARED TO OPERATE ON THE WRONG SIDE BEFORE THE CORRECT SIDE WAS IDENTIFIED

*(**Source:** The Journal of Bone and Joint Surgery, JBJS, 2003)*

form. Ben must live forever with the loss of his sole functioning testicle, and still faces the removal of the diseased testicle that harbors cancer cells.

Wrong site/side, wrong patient/procedure surgery events (WSPE) is a category that includes:

- Operating on or removing the wrong limb or organ
- Operating on the wrong part of the body
- Doing the wrong procedure
- Treating the wrong patient

Some studies state that wrong-site, wrong-side or wrong-patient procedures may occur at a rate as high as 1 in 5,000 surgeries, although other studies put the rate at closer to 1 in 112,994. Even with these varied statistics, an article in the Archives of Surgery (September, 2006) found that wrong-site surgeries may be 20 times more common than previously reported, and current prevention efforts may be inadequate. This study evaluated four databases that hold substantial and confidential reported cases including:

- National Practitioner Data Bank (NPDB) which recorded 5,940 WSPEs including 2,217 wrong-side surgical procedures and 3,723 wrong-treatment/wrong procedure errors over 13 years
- Florida Code 15 mandatory reporting system recorded an average of 75 wrong-side procedures (Florida cases) per year
- American Society of Anesthesiologists (ASA) Closed Claims Project database
- Web-based system for collecting wrong-side, wrong-site, wrong-procedure and wrong-patient adverse events (WSPEs)

Using these four separate databases, the research physicians Samuel C. Seiden and Paul Barach estimated that wrong-site surgery occurs between 1,300 and 2,700 times a year in the U.S.

A study in the Journal of Bone and Joint Surgery (JBJS, 2003) surveyed 1,560 active members of the American Society for Surgery of the Hand (ASSH). Each member was mailed a confidential 29-question survey. More than 1,050 (67 percent) of the surgeons responded.

- 173 surgeons (16 percent) reported they had prepared to operate on the wrong site, but then noticed the error prior to the incision.

- 217 (21 percent) reported performing wrong-site surgery at least once in their career.
- Of an estimated 6,700,000 surgical procedures, 242 were performed at the wrong site, and incidence of one in 27,686 hand procedures.
- The three most common locations of wrong-site surgery were the fingers (153), hands (20) and wrists (21).
- Permanent disability occurred in 21 patients (9 percent).
- 93 cases (38 percent) led to legal action or monetary settlement.

When confidential data is reviewed, frightening results are revealed on wrong-site surgeries. These rates are far above acceptable, no matter what study one believes.

PROTECT YOURSELF IN TODAY'S HEALTHCARE SYSTEM

In 2003, hospitals across the U.S. adopted a new practice called Universal Protocol, largely because of a Joint Commission regulation in response to wrong-site/wrong-side surgeries. Hospitals accredited by the Joint Commission (approximately 80 percent of U.S. hospitals, including military hospitals) are mandated to use a Universal Protocol. The components of an acceptable Universal Protocol include:
- The correct area/side of the body is selected for surgery using available diagnostic tests and examinations.
- The site, side or area to be operated on is marked with an indelible marker. This includes correct limb, body side, or level of the spine for back and neck surgeries.
- Before taking the patient into surgery, a verification process takes place with the patient, including a review of all relevant diagnostic tests, documents and patient information by the pre-surgical team.
- A "time-out" is observed immediately before the procedure begins, to verify all information including correct patient, procedure, site, area and/or side. This involves open communication and active team interaction with the patient for all verification of information.

The Joint Commission inspects records and observes procedures to assure that the Universal Protocol is being used during their onsite inspections, which occur every 18 to 36 months. However, in between inspections, components of the Universal Protocol may be missed or even skipped, depending upon the type of safety systems that are built into a particular hospital's process. It also depends on the human performance of the surgical team. Some surgeons and hospitals have rigid systems in place that mandate tight controls and monitoring of compliance with the Universal Protocol. Other hospitals rely on individual performance by surgeons and surgical teams. These allow for great variation in the Universal Protocols among healthcare systems.

By its own policies, the V.A. hospital was required to obtain informed consent from Ben for the surgery, mark the surgical site and take a "time-out" in the operating room to double-check that doctors were about to perform surgery on the correct site, doing the correct procedure and operating on the correct patient. The V.A. responded to the media and stated they would be changing and enforcing their pre-surgical processes.

Wrong-site/wrong-side surgery is considered a sentinel event. Sentinel describes the term signal, meaning an event is significant enough to trigger a full investigation into the cause of an incident. Sentinel events include any event where a patient dies or has permanent damage. It can also be an event that is significant enough to cause a risk of potential permanent harm or death, such as a wrong-side surgery, or a retained foreign object like an instrument or surgical sponge.

The Joint Commission has a voluntary process for reporting sentinel events, including wrong-site surgeries. It is important to understand that this reporting system is strictly voluntary. Most hospitals do not report sentinel events directly to the Joint Commission, but perform internal root-cause analyses and process changes. A small percentage of hospitals choose to report sentinel events to the Joint Commission. Since no mandatory reporting exists, the exact number of wrong-site surgeries is probably far higher than the Joint Commission sentinel event statistics show on their website.

As mentioned, another identified sentinel event stemming from surgery is the retention of a foreign object. This event is a more common occurrence than wrong-site surgery. Retained objects include surgical sponges, gauze pads, instruments, staples, needles or other items used during a procedure. Although stringent measures are taken to count items, mistakes and human error do occur. A study published in the New England Journal of Medicine (January, 2003) found the risk of retention of a foreign body after surgery significantly increases in emergency surgeries, unplanned changes during a procedure and in obese patients.

When undergoing surgery of any type, it is very important to work closely with your surgeon and the healthcare professionals that will be caring for you. This is particularly true when you are facing a surgery that involves a specific side of the body as well as a specific location, such as spinal or neck surgery. The American College of Surgeons recommends very specific questions to ask your surgeon.

- What is the name of the operation/procedure that will be performed?
- Where, or on what body part, will you be operating?
- Are there any alternatives to the operation?
- What are the risks of this particular procedure?
- What is likely to happen if I don't have the operation?
- Who is in charge of the surgical team?
- Will the correct part of my body be marked before the operation?

NEW SAFEGUARDS

In January 2006 at a children's hospital in California, a child undergoing surgery for a brain tumor suffered an incision on the wrong side of the brain. When an assistant surgeon entered the operating room, the table was turned, allowing for the mistake to occur. After the wrong side of the skull had been opened, the error was discovered and the correct surgery was performed. The child suffered no permanent harm as a result. However, the hospital was cited by the Department of Public Health. The hospital implemented a stringent process in the operating room after this event occurred. No surgical instruments are allowed in the operating room at this children's hospital until a strict Universal Protocol is performed.

The use of the Universal Protocol has no doubt assisted in reducing wrong-site/wrong-side surgeries. Even so, there are studies that show this protocol may only reduce wrong-site/wrong-side surgeries 62 percent of the time. In addition, although there are stringent practices in place for counting instruments and sponges, objects are still retained and people suffer from infections, pain and the need for re-operations as a result. Some hospitals have moved toward technological solutions such as wands and bar coded sponges to track objects retained within the body prior to closing an incision. Starting in October 2008 Medicare will not pay for care when a foreign object is retained during an operation.

After Ben Houghton went public with his story, the chief of staff for the V.A. health system described to the Los Angeles Times that "an electronic rather than a written consent form is now used," meaning that the information in a patient's records goes directly to the form without the risk of a transcription error. And well before the patient is wheeled into the operating room, the surgeon must review the consent form and make sure that the form, the chart and the patient agree on the procedure. Surgeons at the hospital have attended a mandatory time-out workshop on safety and teamwork. It had been planned before the wrong-side error, but the case made it easier to get everyone's attention, according to the V.A. physician.

Even though the V.A. healthcare system has received national attention for patient safety innovations, Ben Houghton has joined the thousands of Americans who are wronged each year by medical errors. Although hundreds of thousands of surgeries are successfully performed each year, it is important to recognize that adverse events like wrong-site surgery and retained foreign objects do occur. Patients must be extremely diligent, participative and alert before and after any surgical procedure. Never take for granted that all safety steps have been performed, and be actively involved in the preparation for surgery, asking many questions, verifying the type and location of the procedure, and reading all consents and paperwork carefully.

Correct Surgery, Correct Body Part: Preventing Surgical Site Errors
- Talk with your surgeon and review carefully and thoroughly what procedure will be performed.
- Neck or spinal surgery involves a specific location. Discuss what level of the spine or neck will be operated on and what approach will the surgeon be using.
- For any surgery involving the hand or foot, specify with your surgeon what will be done. If the surgery involves a fingers or toes, verify with your surgeon which fingers or toes are involved.
- For any surgery involving a specific side of the body, verify with your surgeon the correct side and location.
- When you are being prepared for surgery, review with the nurses the specific procedure you are having performed and the location of the incision.

Before You Sign the Consent Forms
- Read all surgical consents thoroughly.
- Once you have verified the side, site and location of the surgery, carefully review your surgical consent to assure it is accurate.
- Do not sign the consent if any information is incorrect.
  - Insist that the consent be corrected and verify it once again.
- Be sure to verify, understand and sign the surgical consent prior to taking any pre-surgical medication that may impair or interfere with your ability to think or make decisions.

Sentinel Event Monitoring
- Log onto The Joint Commission website for trends on voluntary hospital reporting of Sentinel Events at: www.joint commission.org

CHAPTER 11

THREE LITTLE

In this chapter
- You will learn the devastating impact of preventable medication errors.
    - Medication errors occur when processes in the ordering, delivery and administration of medications within a healthcare system break down.
- Learn about high-alert medications used in hospitals and what precautions you need to take.
- What precautions should hospitals take when administering medications?
- Find out what questions to ask when you or a family member receives medications in the hospital or from a healthcare provider.

Why is it important to know about medication errors?
Each year thousands of hospital patients are the victims of preventable medication errors. In fact, medication errors are the most common type of mistakes made in hospitals and healthcare facilities, sometimes resulting in permanent injury or death. Multiple care delivery system factors in prescribing, ordering, dispensing and administering drugs, including dosage, timing, method, frequency and sound-alike drug names, leave all patients particularly vulnerable to these types of errors.

ANGELS

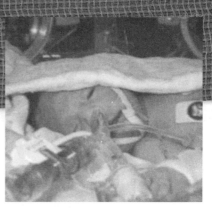

Thursday Dawn Jeffers

It wasn't supposed to be this way, thought Heather Jeffers, as she blinked back tears in front of the news crews that gathered outside her red brick apartment. Seated on a folding chair her mother had carried outside for her, she leaned forward in exhaustion and supported herself against her thighs. Never in her life had she felt so tired and helpless.

Exactly one week ago, Heather had been pregnant and life was ordinary. Her baby wasn't due for at least a month-and-a-half. She still had time to choose a name, make plans. At the time, there was no way she could have imagined how her personal circumstances would collide with a series of tragic errors. Now the results had changed her life forever; her baby died last night.

Heather's mother and sister flanked her, one on each side, as she sat in front of the reporters and photographers. She wore a dark baggy t-shirt and jeans, some of the only clothes that fit so soon after the baby's birth, with a belly still stretched from pregnancy. Had it really been just six days ago? It seemed like months had passed because of all that had happened. Her face was puffy from crying and her eyes were red-rimmed.

What did these news reporters see when they looked at her? Did they understand what really happened? She wondered if they saw just another single mother, another statistic or news story, as if that made her grief any less real or the hospital's mistakes any less horrifying. Although she was acutely aware of the disapproving looks it might draw from others, Heather lit a cigarette with shaking hands, hoping to calm her nerves. She hung her head slightly as her mother and sister comforted her, partially shielding her from the cameras. As she worked to compose herself, she played back the events of the past week in her head.

Wednesday, September 13, 2006

As fall approached the air had cooled off, a huge relief to Heather. The sticky heat and humidity of a southern Indiana summer could always be uncomfortable, but during pregnancy it had felt oppressive. It weighed her down, and made the baby she was carrying feel twice as heavy. Edging into her eighth month now, Heather had reached the point so many expectant mothers know all too well; she was anxious for the pregnancy to be over and done, and have her baby girl with her. Just another seven weeks to go, she reminded herself, and this would be behind her.

Parenthood wasn't going to be easy, Heather knew that. Her due date in November would be here soon, and she worried about how to make ends meet. Raising a baby alone as a single parent would be a challenge, but she had a supportive mother who was close by. That made her luckier than many young mothers. She tried to focus on the positive, getting things ready for her new daughter, and on the anticipation of wondering what her baby would be like. That helped her get beyond any fears about the future.

With summer behind her, Heather had more energy. She began making a nest for the baby, and felt like getting out of her small apartment more often. She noticed how active the baby had been lately, kicking and pushing against the walls of her small, confined world. Maybe the baby felt more like getting out too, and the thought amused her.

The sensation came on unexpectedly while she was walking, a strong cramping that seized her hips and abdomen. It caught her off guard, causing Heather to hold her breath for a moment. She rode the wave of pain to its peak and relaxed as it subsided, only to have another one several minutes later. Although it was only September, she realized what was happening. It's too soon, she thought. The baby isn't ready yet; I'm not ready yet. I haven't even picked out a name. I haven't packed a bag.

Alone and frightened, Heather called her mother, Joanna. She would know what to do. "Mom, I think I'm having labor pains. I'm scared," Heather's voice quavered over the phone.

"What do you mean? This is way too early for that," her mother dismissed the possibility. She assumed her daughter was simply nervous and worrying over nothing. It must be the jitters of a first-time mother. But Heather was insistent.

Joanna reassured her daughter that it was probably false labor. "It happens to everyone. There's no reason to panic," she tried to calm Heather. "If it makes you feel better I'll take you to the hospital and they can check you out there, just to be safe."

Within minutes, Joanna arrived to find Heather more uncomfortable than she expected. The short distance to the hospital might as well have been across the state, as far as Heather was concerned. It felt like forever as the pains became closer and more intense, but she still wondered if she was overreacting. My mom's probably right, she thought, it must be false labor and I'm going to the hospital for nothing. They'll say everything is okay, and then I'll go home feeling embarrassed.

Once in the obstetrics unit at the hospital, it was clear that Heather's labor was for real and it was a force in motion. There would be no stopping it. "I'm only 32 or 33 weeks," she told the staff between contractions, as they prepared her for labor and delivery. The baby has been so strong and active, Heather thought, she'll be fine.

Heather felt confident that everything would be fine, even though the baby was coming early. This hospital was well-known locally for their wonderful obstetrics care and neonatal unit. Now she was in good hands.

Thursday, September 14

In the early hours before dawn on Thursday, September 14, Heather delivered her baby girl. She caught a brief glimpse of her daughter, slippery and glistening in the reflection from the lights, as they held the baby up for one fleeting moment before whisking her away. "She's so tiny," Heather said with awe, unprepared for how small her premature baby would actually be. She had never seen a preemie before. With no name chosen until now, Heather decided to call her Thursday Dawn.

From across the room she could see the nurses surrounding Thursday, obscuring her view of the baby. They worked quietly but quickly, and Heather wished she knew what mysterious things they were doing with her daughter. "Four pounds, six ounces," she heard someone in the group call out the baby's weight. After that the nurses spoke in muffled tones, but Heather could pick up some of what they were saying, and it alarmed her.

"Her Apgars don't look good."

"Her breathing isn't good. We'll have to intubate."

"Notify NICU to receive an admission."

Heather tried to hear more, but her head felt fuzzy from the medication. With her mouth dry and her skin moist with sweat, she was spent from the delivery and would have to trust that Thursday was in the best hands. There was nothing she could do for her. A nurse assured Heather she could see the baby later when they had her stabilized, telling her the NICU, or neonatal intensive care unit, was a safe place with everything her daughter needed.

The next time Heather saw her daughter was in the NICU that evening, where they had taken her so quickly after the birth. Earlier in the day a doctor had explained to her why Thursday was there, that her lungs were still undeveloped and she couldn't breathe well on her own. Soon, when her lungs matured and she gained some weight, they promised Thursday could go home.

A nurse escorted Heather into the NICU and led her to where Thursday lay sleeping in an incubator. The enclosed structure reminded her of a large fish tank, but with arm-holes big enough for people to reach in and care for the baby. Nothing prepared Heather to see her baby in a glass box where she couldn't hold her. A tube was coming out of Thursday's navel and she was connected to a respirator. Sensors attached to her torso monitored her tiny body's functions. Periodically she would make a sudden jerky movement that reminded Heather she was real.

Heather felt overwhelmed by the sights and smells in the NICU, and by the fatigue from giving birth earlier in the day. As she looked for something to lean against, the nurse carried over a chair for her to sit on and placed it next to the incubator.

Throughout the room there were beds like Thursday's, as well as some that were flat and open with glass sides for the tiniest preemies. She could hear beeps coming from one of the machines attached to Thursday. An alarm on a device across the room startled her, and another nurse quickly shut it off and checked on the infant next to it.

The nurse stood by Heather and patiently explained the purpose of all the tubes. "This one in her mouth is helping her breathe until her lungs are stronger. This tube," she pointed to Thursday's navel, "is giving her fluid and medicine through an IV line. Her belly button gives us a perfect place for that—better than trying to put an IV in her tiny veins." Heather felt tears welling up in her eyes unexpectedly, and seeing this, the nurse silently rubbed her shoulder. This first visit was always so hard for parents, thought the nurse. No one envisions their child spending the first days of life in a place like this, a place where progress is measured in grams and cubic centimeters—small but important victories.

Heather sat next to Thursday and tried to memorize every detail of her baby's face and body; her delicate, wrinkled skin covered with soft fuzz, her feathery eyelashes, and the tiny fingernail buds that hadn't really grown in yet. In that moment, she was completely absorbed in her daughter and forgot any of her own physical discomfort from the birth. The staff allowed her to reach into the incubator and gently touch Thursday, and the baby immediately grasped her finger. She's a fighter, Heather thought.

Later that evening, a doctor stopped by Heather's room to tell her that Thursday had a good chance of doing well, and might be ready to go home in just a month. She began to feel more optimistic about the situation; the baby was getting such good care. For the first time since the birth she allowed herself to rest, but Heather found it hard to sleep; she couldn't stop thinking about her baby, and it felt the same as falling in love.

Friday, September 15

Several new moms were in the NICU on Friday when Heather came to visit her daughter. The NICU became a central gathering place for these parents, like the post office or coffee shop in a small town. While spending time with their child they would meet others in their situation. They shared stories and traded information, bonded with their new friends by a common experience that only they could understand.

Chairs were conveniently stationed around the nursery, and as she sat down Heather scanned the room, taking in the other mothers and mentally comparing Thursday with the other preemies. Her gaze landed on another mom seated next to the smallest baby she had ever seen. The infant was in one of the open glass-walled beds for the most premature patients, a radiant warmer. I wonder how far along she was when her baby was born, Heather thought, and decided to ask.

"I was only at 25 weeks when I delivered Emmery," answered Evie Miller, the baby's mother. "I call her my little jewel. My birthstone is an Emerald but I didn't want to call her that, so I named her Emmery. She was born yesterday, and she only weighed a little over a pound."

The same birthday, thought Heather, and she told Evie the story of how she named her baby Thursday Dawn. Another young woman entered the NICU as Heather spoke, and leaned over a radiant warmer bed across the room. "Hi D'myia, it's Mommy. I missed you last night," she cooed as she stroked the baby.

Evie already knew this mother, and introduced her as Whittney. Heather asked how long her baby had been in the NICU. Four days, she was told. "She was just one pound, four ounces when she was born, but she's already gained two ounces," Whittney boasted, looking very proud. If these babies who were far more premature could do this well, Heather thought, Thursday should have few problems.

Late Friday evening the hospital staff arrived for the night shift, and the transfer of duties began as it did on countless other shift changes. There was always an overlap, as those who were leaving the hospital filled in their replacements on any need-to-know information. The twenty-four hour nature of the place created a constant ebb and flow of vital personnel and information, rotating in rhythmic cycles around the clock.

Peter, a pharmacy technician, arrived fifteen minutes early, just as he always did, so he would have time for a cup of coffee before he checked in. A tall, affable man with thinning hair and a pleasant disposition, he didn't mind the late shift; it worked well with his schedule and, as a rule, he could get things done with fewer interruptions. After 25 years on the job he was not only efficient, but he had seniority as well, and could get the shifts he wanted more easily.

Around 11:00 that night, the pharmacy received a standard order from the NICU for routine drugs they needed to stock. The pharmacist printed an invoice form, or pick ticket, that the pharmacy technician takes back to the drug inventory and uses to fill the order. Peter took the pick ticket to the warehouse and began to fill the order. He would then pack and deliver it on his own, stocking the automated medicine dispensing cabinet himself. Looking at the ticket he noticed it was for the NICU, and smiled as he thought about the babies there. Some were so small they could almost fit in his hand.

Saturday, September 16
The NICU order called for 25 vials of Hep-lock, located on shelf 1-A in the pharmacy warehouse. Finding the Hep-lock, Peter reached up with his long arms and pulled a box of 25 vials off the shelf. He loaded them into a tote used to transport drugs and left to deliver the order.

He entered the NICU, and as he passed the nurses on duty he said hello with a friendly nod and a smile. At 1:17 a.m., Peter signed into the automated drug cabinet using his pass code and safely stocked the pre-loaded vials where they belonged, then left quietly so he wouldn't disturb the quiet atmosphere of the nursery.

One of the NICU nurses, Sam, was scrubbing her hands and preparing to put on gloves. Sam liked working on Friday nights, because for the hospital administrators the weekend had already begun. There were fewer administrative housekeeping duties that had little to do with hands-on nursing, and it was usually calmer than a weeknight. That meant fewer distractions that took her away from patient care, the part of the job she really enjoyed.

They had full staffing tonight, she noticed, so there would be extra time to make sure the babies in her care were comfortable. She surveyed her small patients and noted everything looked good. None of the infants were lying on wires or IV lines and they all seemed content. Checking Emmery Miller's ventilator settings, tubes and lines, Sam saw that she was sleeping soundly. She listened carefully to the baby's heart and lungs before moving on to the next child.

After returning from her dinner break at 3:00 in the morning, Sam checked once again on the sleeping Emmery and saw that she was stable. Jennifer, the nurse who covered for Sam during the break, could leave for dinner now. "Nothing's changed with my babies,"

Jennifer said matter-of-factly as she left the NICU and headed for the cafeteria, "and I already flushed their IV lines."

Now it was time for Sam to flush the IV lines on her preemies. She prepared to inject a small pre-measured dose of Heparin, a blood thinning agent, into the IV ports attached to the infants' navels. This kept the vein clear, and the IV unobstructed by clotting blood. During a 12-hour shift, the nurses might flush the lines on each baby up to four times. Tonight they were so settled and at ease, it wouldn't take long at all.

Sam walked over to the automated drug cabinet and punched in her pass code. She reached in for a Hep-lock bottle with the familiar blue label and removed it, then carefully closed the cabinet. Preparing the IV flush, she carefully cleaned little Emmery's IV port with a sterile alcohol pad and slowly infused the heparin into he baby's line. Then she repeated the process for the next infant.

A Saturday morning shift change went without incident, as Sam and the other nurses went through the same rituals as they had the night before when they came on duty. The staff handed off information to those coming in and made a final check on their little babies before leaving their posts. Everything seemed in order.

By Saturday afternoon, the nurses noticed something had gone terribly wrong with many of the infants in the NICU. Some of the babies were bleeding from the IV ports in their navels, as well as from their noses. They had blood in their urine and purplish-red bruising under their skin. Lethargic and gravely ill, a number of tiny preemies had entered a downward spiral they might not pull out of. They were fading before everyone's eyes in the most awful way imaginable, bleeding to death internally. The gnawing question was, why? Doctors and nurses were desperate to find clues to what had happened.

The NICU was in a state of alert as medical staff began their desperate efforts to save the affected infants. But it was already too late for at least two of the little girls. Small and weak, premature babies were among the most vulnerable patients in the hospital, defenseless against everything.

That same day, Heather had enjoyed a wonderful afternoon visiting with her family and little Thursday. The discomfort from the birth had eased, and she was looking forward to a good night's sleep before she left the hospital to go home the following day.

As evening approached, a commotion outside the door to Heather's room startled her as she rested.

Someone was screaming, "You won't stop CPR until you tell me the name of the nurse who did this to my baby! What's her name?" It sounded like Evie's voice.

Those in the NICU had quickly discovered the wrenching truth; a massive overdose of heparin had caused the life-threatening internal hemorrhages. Six babies had received a potent adult-strength dose of the drug, and three of them had received it more than one time. The nurses on duty never realized they were injecting the fatal doses. Peter, the pharmacy technician, never realized he stocked the wrong dosages in the drug cabinet; the bottles heparin and Hep-lock looked nearly identical to one another.

Heather quickly went to the door. She saw a loud, angry group of people in the hall, and several security guards were pulling someone toward a room off to the side. Although she only saw her back for a moment, Heather knew it was Evie, still wearing her robe and hospital gown. The crowd of people (Evie's relatives, she thought) followed behind, hurrying into the room before the door shut tight. Heather heard muffled yelling and crying from inside the door, but she couldn't make out what they were saying. She felt a gnawing, sick feeling in the pit of her stomach, like something bad was about to happen and her body knew it before her head.

11%

PERCENTAGE OF MEDICATION ERRORS INVOLVING DANGEROUS HIGH-ALERT MEDICATIONS, SUCH AS HEPARIN, MORPHINE, INSULIN, POTASSIUM CHLORIDE AND CHEMOTHERAPY AGENTS

5.7%
(nearly 6 out of every 100)

PERCENTAGE OF MEDICATION ORDERS FOR PEDIATRIC PATIENTS THAT CONTAIN ERRORS

As Heather turned back to walk toward her room, she sensed being followed. A chill ran up her spine, ending at the nape of her neck. She spun around and was surprised to find a group of important looking people standing in front of her. Confused, she wondered what these people would be doing here on a Saturday night—talking to her. Pulling her robe more tightly around her, Heather shivered a little again, and her teeth chattered slightly as if she was out in the cold. Something was headed her way and she was powerless to stop it, or to even get out of its path.

Finally, one of the men began speaking, "Ms. Jeffers, I'm the hospital CEO." The others with him were attorneys and doctors, but Heather didn't hear any names as they introduced themselves. All the blood seemed to rush from her head and she couldn't concentrate. She heard the voices, but couldn't comprehend the words. Only random pieces of what they said made it through the gauzy filter of shock.

"Accident...heparin...critical...sorry."

Now Heather heard her mother yelling, "What do you mean? What's wrong with Thursday?" Joanna's voice became increasingly shrill and hysterical. "What did you do to her?" she demanded.

"We need to transfer your baby to the children's hospital," another man in a suit turned and addressed Heather. "They can treat her condition there. That's her best chance."

Her legs seemed to liquefy as she tried to steady herself against the doorway of her hospital room. Like a fuzzy picture that comes into focus when it's adjusted, for the first time she saw the full view of what was happening. Evie's baby was dead, and now these people were here to see her about Thursday.

Heather felt like she was having a nightmare and wished she would wake up, but no nightmare could be this vivid, this detailed. Suddenly aware that she was holding her breath, Heather felt something rising inside and knew that if she took in air, a primal noise would escape from her. She leaned against her mother's chest and let herself take a deep breath, and a long, mournful wail came out as she exhaled. Then her mother's arms folded around her and Heather sobbed.

Sunday, September 17

The scope of the tragedy and insight into the chain of events continued to grow on Sunday. After Heather learned about Thursday's condition, she heard that D'Myia, Whittney's baby, died just as Emmery Miller had. Three other babies had received only one heparin injection instead of two, and were expected to survive.

Little Thursday was now at the local children's hospital, where doctors were trying to stop the bleeding and make her blood clot with medications. Thursday was bigger than the two infants who died, and Heather used that fact as a hook on which to hang her hopes.

By Sunday afternoon, the busy hospital had as many rumors as it had beds. In the initial absence of information about what happened, the staff drew their own conclusions about the events. The buzz flowed through the corridors and rooms with the same energy as an electrical current. Hospital administrators quickly organized a series of special staff briefings for that afternoon, in an effort to address concerns and squelch rumors. It seemed almost every employee had questions about the incident.

"Are the other babies going to die?"

"Who was the tech? Who are the nurses?"

"Are they going to get fired? I heard they were sent home early."

The devastation radiated outward from the original event like ripples in a pond, spreading anguish to everyone who was directly or indirectly involved: victims, families, nurses, doctors, technicians, chaplains. It was difficult to see where the impact would end.

Sam and Jennifer from the NICU, along with other nurses who had been on duty at the time, had to be escorted home by security guards for their own protection. So did the pharmacy technician, Peter. They received death threats and feared for their safety. After years of providing care and compassion to patients, each one was emotionally ravaged and guilt-ridden over what had occurred. At home on leave from their jobs, the hospital offered chaplains and counselors to help them cope with the nightmarish sequence of events. But in private moments, they endlessly replayed the scenario in their own minds and pondered how this could have happened.

Reporters swarmed the hospital in an effort to get interviews or discover a new lead. The hospital president and CEO planned a news conference for 5:00 that day, so until then the press would be camped out, hoping more information would be revealed at the end of the day.

The CEO began the conference by reading a statement for the media. "It is with deep regret we report that two premature infants died and four other infants were affected Saturday evening, Sept. 16, in our hospital's newborn intensive care unit, where our most fragile patients receive care. It appears, preliminarily, that vials with an inappropriately high level of heparin, a blood-thinning agent, were mistakenly administered to six infants in place of those with the lower, correct dose.

"We are currently conducting a through investigation of all the facts . . ."

He finished his statement with a reference to the victims and their families. "This is a tragic event and our thoughts and prayers are extended to the families. When something like this occurs, we are all affected from the nurses at the bedside to the CEO. All of us are in healthcare because of our unwavering commitment to helping people, and this incident hurts us all. As we move forward with the investigation, we will continue to provide more information as we learn more."

At the children's hospital with her baby, Heather didn't see the news conference. It wouldn't have mattered; everything she needed to know was contained in the incubator in front of her. Someone had hurt her baby, whether they meant to or not, but at least Thursday was still alive.

Monday, September 18
Heavy rain fell all day, adding to the atmosphere of gloom. Heather's emotions fluctuated between fear and hope, and they rose and fell with each assessment of her baby's condition. The doctors told her Thursday was in critical condition and had yet to show any significant signs of improvement, but no one was giving up on her. They were still giving her medication in an attempt to counteract the heparin.

When she went home to rest and change her clothes Heather saw news accounts about the deaths of Emmery and D'myia on television. A reporter on News 13 caught her attention when she talked about

Whittney. "Whittney says on Saturday a hospital official called and told her medical staff made a mistake by giving her daughter an overdose of heparin. That overdose proved lethal. Whittney says the hospital's apology doesn't help her understand how this could have happened," the reporter finished.

There was Whittney being interviewed on camera. "I feel like whoever the nurse was on call should have known what she was doing and how much my baby should have," she told the reporter. Heather agreed with what Whittney said. How could they call this a mistake, as if it was something trivial like dialing a wrong phone number? The word didn't fit.

Heather's thoughts were interrupted when she heard the telephone. Her mother, Joanna, who was there waiting to take her back to the hospital, answered it after a few rings. "It's someone from the hospital," she called to Heather in her bedroom. "He's asking to talk to you. Says he wants to discuss how they might help you, and see how you're doing."

"I don't want to hear anything he has to say," Heather yelled back from her room, as she brushed her hair furiously before pulling it back in a hair band. She didn't have time for their excuses right now. She had to get back to her baby.

Tuesday, September 19

Every time the phone rang now, Heather wondered who it would be. Reporters, hospital executives, lawyers—by Monday night she began using her answering machine to screen calls. Right now she didn't know who to speak to, so it was easier to avoid almost everyone. It was hard to know who to trust or why they were really calling.

Her mother was there with her again on Tuesday night. Joanna didn't think Heather should be trying to drive herself anywhere right now, between the recovery from the birth and the emotional upset. So she was here at her disposal. There wasn't much she could do about the situation right now, but she could do that much. She could be there, and make sure her own little girl was safe.

It was getting late in the evening when the phone rang again. Joanna and Heather let it go to the answering machine, but both raced to grab it when they realized it was the children's hospital trying to reach them. Heather picked up the phone, breathless. "Hello, hello. I'm here," she nearly yelled into the handset, afraid they would think she wasn't there and hang up. Joanna saw Heather grimace and her chin tremble. "Mom," she cried, as she clenched her eyes shut against the tears and reached for Joanna.

The ICU at Riley was able to keep Thursday going until Heather and Joanna arrived. A nurse seated Heather in a big, white rocking chair with blue cushions, located in the corner of a small, quiet room decorated with pastel flowers. It was softly lit and homey. A doctor unhooked Thursday from the respirator, IV and monitors that had been her constant companions since birth, and the nurse wrapped her in a homemade patchwork quilt before presenting her to Heather.

For the first time since she was born, Heather could hold her baby girl and rock her. She hummed to Thursday as she leaned over and breathed in the baby's scent, trying to commit it to memory. As she stroked Thursday's cheek with the back of her hand, silent tears rolled down her face in a continuous trickle, leaving wet spots where they fell on the quilt. Heather pulled back the quilt from around the baby's ankles so she could gently rub her tiny feet. After a few more minutes had passed, the nurse came back with a stethoscope and listened for the baby's heart and respiration. Thursday was gone. Heather held the baby to her chest and continued to rock for awhile.

Wednesday, September 20
Here was Heather before the cameras and reporters in front of her apartment. Joanna told Heather this would be an opportunity to tell their story and warn others that this could happen to them. Her mother had spoken with the TV stations and newspapers, and said she would agree to a news conference here, today. Joanna promised she would do most of the talking so Heather didn't have to.

The hospital contacted Heather again today, and wanted to pay for the funeral expenses for Thursday and the other babies. They offered to pay for counseling, too, and said they recommended it. When the hospital talked about providing restitution Heather thought about what an odd word it is, like you could restore a person, even though she knew that's not what it meant. She thought about last night with Thursday, and underneath the pretty quilt, the red and purple marks that covered her baby's body and gave away how she died. Buried beneath her pain and sorrow there was a mound of anger pushing up, and she knew it would come to the surface soon.

Joanna made a statement and answered a few questions from some reporters, but when Heather tried to speak, she could only turn to her mother and cry. "They killed my baby. Why?"

Heather, Evie and Whittney never imagined that their paths would collide in such a tragic series of events. Their three little girls, conceived within a few months of one another, were born early, but all were expected to be home by Christmas. Instead, they were taken too soon. The mothers of these angels will try to put their lives back together again, but on their babies' birthdays each September they will remember, and wonder what their daughters might have become.

This journey should have had a happy ending, but the path was lined with fatal points. With millions of medications administered everyday in hospitals, these points can occur at any stage in the care process, and take everyone involved down a terrible path. Those who work at the hospital where this occurred are shell shocked, and describe this as their 9/11.

At 33 weeks gestation, little Thursday was too premature to take in nourishment through breast feeding or a bottle, so she had to receive nourishment through an intravenous line (IV). The blood vessel from her umbilical cord provided a perfect route for these IV fluids, but the umbilical blood vessels can become clogged with drying blood. To keep the vein open, a tiny concentration of the drug heparin, an anticoagulant, is injected into the rubber port of the IV. Larger adult dosages of heparin, 1,000 times stronger than the infant dosage, are used to prevent deadly blood clots that could cause heart attack or stroke in adults.

Nationally, heparin is listed in a group of medications with a *high alert* warning, because the consequences of an incorrect dosage can be dire and at times fatal. Other medications in this high alert category include insulin, morphine, chemotherapy drugs, potassium, and electrolyte solutions.

For over a decade, hospitals have been installing automated medication dispensing cabinets that contain numerous small drawers. These drawers are designed to organize and categorize medications into individual compartments. This design helps to avoid random mix-ups of medications that were previously stored in containers on shelves in the hospital units. The drawers are secured by computerized locks and accessed by a password or code, allowing a nurse to select medications intended for a particular patient.

Yet these cabinets may provide a false sense of security. Hospital pharmacies are responsible for stocking automated cabinets with medications, and in many facilities the orders are filled and stocked by a pharmacy technician or pharmacist without a double-check.

A recent survey of hospitals by the Institute for Safe Medication Practices (ISMP) found that only 11 percent of the drugs placed in medication cabinets were always verified by a second person.

A cascade of flaws in the healthcare system caused the tragic mistake that, ultimately, took the lives of three babies. Two similar-looking medications were confused with one another by several healthcare professionals. A manual system with multiple hand-offs from beginning to end, and lacking electronic safeguards, was used to process the medications.

The sequence of events occurred in a deadly but logical progression, each step flowing from the last. A technician with more than 25 years of experience made a crucial error in stocking of a high alert medication, and experienced nurses believed they were giving the proper dosage of the correct medication. This was primarily because

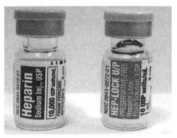

Vials similar to those confused.

there were no technological safeguards in place, allowing for human error to perpetuate at multiple fatal points because there were so many similarities between the packaging of the two drugs (see picture of vials):

1 in 25

NICU PATIENTS THAT
HAVE A MEDICATION
ERROR OCCUR TO
THEM

- Look-alike drug boxes were stored alphabetically and in close proximity in the pharmacy warehouse.
- The boxes containing both heparin doses are similar in size, color and markings.
- Both boxes contained individual vials of heparin.
- The heparin bottles are identical in size and shape for both dosages.
- The pharmaceutical company failed to build in safeguards in order to distinguish similar looking bottles with significantly different doses.
- Both heparin bottles are made from the same color of plastic.
- The labels on both bottles are similar; one is baby blue and one is primary blue.

- The lids are similar, with only slight variation when looking down at the bottle top.
- Both labels contain the same first three letters—heparin and hep-lock.
- The nurses never had access to full-dose heparin and wouldn't have expected it to be there; the pharmacy only stocked the NICU cabinet with hep-lock for infant dosage.

Nurses are taught a system of checks and balances for administering medication called the five rights:
- right patient
- right drug
- right dose
- right route, and
- right time

Every time a medication is given, the five rights are to be carried out, even when administering an aspirin. While this practice has been taught to nurses for decades, it's clearly not a fail-proof system. It relies heavily on human memory instead of failsafe technologies. Although important, it is still a weak protection method for keeping patients safe, and it failed miserably in this situation. An opportunity for error can occur if even one of the five rights is omitted at any time.

But even when all five rights are carried out, this system of checks could still fail, as demonstrated by one last fatal point. The wrong dosage was withdrawn from the original "wrong" vials and injected multiple times. Why? It happened because people conform

14%

PERCENTAGE OF HEPARIN RELATED MEDICATION ERRORS THAT RESULT IN SERIOUS PATIENT HARM

31%

PERCENTAGE OF MEDICATION ERRORS THAT RESULT FROM ADMINISTRATION OF THE WRONG DOSE FOR A PRESCRIBED DRUG

11%

NUMBER OF TIMES DRUGS PLACED IN AUTOMATED MEDICATION DISPENSING CABINETS VERIFIED BY A SECOND PERSON

10%

ESTIMATED
PERCENTAGE OF U.S.
HOSPITALS THAT USE
BARCODE TECHNOLOGY
FOR ALL MEDICATIONS

to routine patterns and expect those patterns to repeat each time. Because all the nurses routinely flushed IV ports with low-dose heparin, they followed a blind path. Once again, people are creatures of habit, and it perpetuated the error.

It may be tempting to cast blame on the nurses or the pharmacy technician for the tragic events that caused the babies' deaths, but it's vital to look beyond this. Both the patients and the healthcare professionals were victims of system failures, leading to a cascade of missteps. Yes, people failed to keep the infants safe, but broken systems were more at fault than the people who were involved.

Today in healthcare, human error is a substantial contributing factor in preventable adverse events. In early aviation, human error led to many aircraft disasters. Pilot errors were common. Without fail-resistant engineering technology and multiple back-up systems, too much rested on the pilots.

Technology, such as bar coding removes the sole reliance on memory, and essentially performs an "electronic five rights" every time, for every drug, for every patient. Bar coding coordinates the identification of the patient by their ID band, the nurse's ID scan, and each drug bar code scan. If the first NICU nurse had scanned the three bar codes, then she would have immediately noticed the wrong dosage, alerting everyone and stopping the fatal injections.

85%

AVERAGE DECLINE IN
MEDICATION ERRORS
WHEN A HOSPITAL
USES BARCODE
TECHNOLOGY TO
DISPENSE AND
ADMINISTER DRUGS TO
PATIENTS

IT'S HAPPENED BEFORE - IT'LL HAPPEN AGAIN

While it's tragic that this type of error occurred, it is far more tragic that it will happen again before the broken systems are fixed. Dr. Albert Wu from Johns Hopkins Hospital, one of the authors of the 2006 Institute of Medicine (IOM) report, spoke about the Indiana event and stated that this is "depressingly normal."

In February, 2002, little baby Gianni was born in a New York hospital and admitted to the NICU. Due to a miscalculation, a fatal dose of potassium chloride was given to Gianni which immediately stopped his heart. The most dreadful part of this tragedy is that seven years earlier, in the same hospital, in the same neonatal intensive care unit, a baby girl named Petra received a ten-fold overdose of morphine. Petra went into respiratory arrest and, fortunately, she was resuscitated and survived the mistake. In the case of baby Petra, the reaction was to cast a wide net of blame on the nurses and doctors, and regulators told the hospital to create a disciplinary policy. Unfortunately, none of these mandates called for safer systems which would have stopped the error that, seven years later, took little Gianni's life.

As mentioned in the Prologue, Dennis Quaid and his wife were also adversely affected by an unintentional, but potentially fatal heparin overdose given to their young twins.

PROTECT YOURSELF IN TODAY'S HEALTHCARE SYSTEM

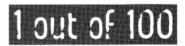

PEDIATRIC MEDICATION ORDERS LIKELY TO RESULT IN ADVERSE DRUG EVENTS

Putting preventative measures in place at hospitals will save lives in the future. Hospitals can take multiple steps to prevent and mitigate such catastrophic errors by addressing medication care processes in place; such as:
- Mandatory special storage of high alert medications.
- A mandatory second check by at least one other pharmacist or technician prior to filling orders, especially for high-alert medications.
- Installation of bar code scanners to read drug label bar codes, electronically ensuring the five rights are performed on every drug for every patient.
- Electronic technology for prescribing and recording patient

medications.

- High alert medication warnings for drugs that carry greater risks.
- Hospital rounds in intensive care units for pharmacists to check medications that are stocked and being administered.
- Improvements in look-alike medication labels and packaging by the drug companies.
- Elimination of high-dose heparin in hospitals that treat children or newborns (much smaller doses of heparin can be purchased for use).
- Use of saline solution as an alternative to heparin for flushing IV lines and keeping veins open (some studies show this method is just as effective).

Many of these safety steps were implemented immediately after the tragedy at the hospital that had this unfortunate incident happen to them, but today all this still can't reverse the damage done. This hospital will continue to be diligent and may avoid this error in the future, but no hospital in the country can guarantee this sequence of events will not occur. Don't think for a moment that the national press coverage about the error at this hospital has caused other hospitals to implement changes, and avoid the same types of mistakes. And don't think that other hospitals in the U.S. have not given the wrong dose of a dangerous drug, or had a very close call. Errors occur at some of the nation's most highly-regarded hospitals. Excellence does not mean infallibility.

Protecting yourself and your family requires a willingness to speak up and ask questions about the medications and treatments your doctor prescribes. Healthcare professionals should never resent honest questions about the medications they administer. As a patient you need to:

- Find out what safeguards your hospital uses to prevent medication errors.
- Know what medications are being administered and why; ask the nurse or physician.
- Immediately report any adverse changes in condition that occur after receiving a medication.

- If something about a medication or dosage doesn't seem right, speak up; never automatically assume the hospital staff is right and you are wrong.

WHEN AND HOW WILL THE HEALTHCARE SYSTEM "LEARN"?

To say that the healthcare industry is in a sorry state and needs help to better "understand and learn" from errors committed in the past would be an understatement. Call it coincidence or a call-to-action message, but just as this manuscript was going to the publisher for printing the exact same medication error that occurred in Indiana repeated itself at a hospital in Los Angeles, California. This time the two babies affected were the Dennis Quaid twins. Naturally, the media coverage on this unfortunate event has been heavy. Why should this be the case? After all, medical errors have now been recognized as the fourth leading cause of death in the US.

The Quaid medical error that occurred 14 months after the Indiana heparin incident highlights the fact that the industry just did not "learn" despite wide availability of root cause analysis and recommendations. This question must be asked: When will hospitals learn to change their systems that result in preventable medical errors? When the now infamous report *"To Err is Human"* was released in 1999 by the Institute of Medicine (IOM), many healthcare professionals felt that at last, a major report substantiated what many knew all too well—people were being harmed by preventable medical errors. Clearly, it is well documented that existing healthcare delivery systems are broken. Although the health industry has toiled to change these systems since then, enough has NOT been enough!

Fatal Care has taken you through an admittedly unpleasant journey. We've shown how individual lives are impacted by preventable medical errors, and some of the steps that you as consumers can take to better protect yourselves from preventable "harm."

With the occurrence of an almost identical error in another Neonatal Intensive Care Unit at a world renowned hospital, there are no more excuses. Both the pharmaceutical company and the hospital

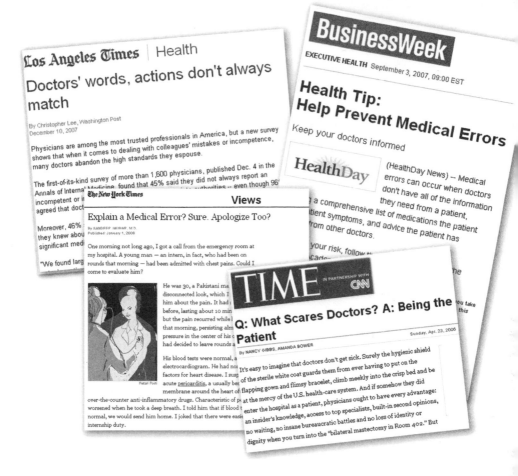

need to take a serious look at why they did not heed the warning and the lessons learned from the Indiana babies incident. These cascades of deadly errors must stop. No more excuses, no more blaming broken healthcare systems.

To mitigate the Quaid case, multiple and stark warnings should have been heeded from the Indiana event. The pharmaceutical company should have made major changes to their labeling and warning systems, regulators should have alerted hospitals to potential danger from this error and hospitals should have built safeguards to stop this preventable error. How many NICU are still vulnerable to this deadly error?

The health industry is not listening; it is not learning. Why didn't the pharmaceutical company change the labeling to red, orange or yellow on the low dose Heparin boxes and vials? They have had longer than a year to make this change. There are no more explanations. Fortunately, for Dennis and Kimberly, the twins are recovering, hopefully with no residual harm, unlike the three Indiana mothers that will never again hold their baby girls. The next family may not be as fortunate. If this runaway train of preventable medical errors does not stop, no baby, no child, no adult will be safe from becoming a new victim of today's fractured health system.

- Be involved in every aspect of your care—play an active part with your healthcare team.
- Use the Internet to research your condition, common errors, effect of medications—become empowered and know your options.
- Speak up, ask questions, and get informed.
- If you have a family member in the hospital who cannot speak up, ask questions for them and be informed.
- Talk to your doctors and nurses daily.
- Learn about any medication prescribed for you or a family member and ask:
  - What are the medication(s) for?
  - What are the side effects of the medication(s)?
  - How long do you need to take the medication(s)?
  - Do any of the medications ordered or prescribed interact with other medication(s) you might be taking?
- To learn more about medication safety go to the Institute for Safe Medication Practices at: www.ismp.org

WHAT ARE HIGH ALERT MEDICATIONS?

Most medications are safe when used correctly, but some drugs have a greater risk of serious injury when they are misused. These are called *high alert drugs*. They have many valuable uses in treating patients; however, if an error occurs with these medications it can cause significant harm. It is good to be aware of high alert medications and make sure proper precautions are used when they are administered. Learn why you need a specific medication and ask questions about how it will be used. The top 5 high alert medications are:

- Heparin—a blood thinner.
- Morphine—a narcotic.
- Potassium Chloride—used to treat certain electrolyte

imbalances.

- Insulin—used mainly for diabetes mellitus to control blood sugar.
- Chemotherapy (cancer fighting) solutions—used to treat different types of cancers.

EPILOGUE

The State of Healthcare Today

The numbers are staggering. Each year, about 98,000 Americans die due to preventable medical errors. Since 2006, the Institute for Healthcare Improvement (IHI) has committed itself to protecting patients from five million incidents of fatal medical harm over a two-year period. This epidemic needs attention now. We launched an early version of www.fatalcare.com in the spring of 2007 and were astounded about the raw number and vitriolic responses received from every corner of the country.

When you reflect on the stories in this book, which unfortunately are all true, even the most callous amongst us begins to realize the gravity and overwhelming impact that preventable medical errors have on those affected. There are common threads which link the stories together and paint a portrait of our current "fractured" health system. In each, it is clear the healthcare consumer, i.e. the patient, was in the dark about the inherent dangers present within the healthcare system when they entered it. As a result, each one of the patients suffered significantly, in some cases with fatal consequences.

Ask a question of yourself. If you were placed in any of these situations, do you know enough to prevent a similar outcome? The point of this book isn't to scare; rather it's to arm the healthcare consumer with knowledge that things can go wrong. How you, the informed healthcare consumer responds, is up to you.

Regardless of any future improvements, technological innovations or additional safety measures, errors will still occur within health systems that we have come to trust. The healthcare industry can limit, but not eliminate risks and errors. This means that even as new policies, technology and equipment make healthcare safer, the patient also has a responsibility to help mitigate errors and must take the initiative to be informed, which leads to being empowered. Consequently, the healthcare industry must provide more open access to safety information and data so consumers can do their part.

Although there is a groundswell for publicly accessible, high-quality data, the volume and actual value of consumer safety data is still very limited. Currently, it remains easier for the consumer to log onto a website and find ratings on cars and clothes dryers, than to find transparent and meaningful safety and quality information about hospitals and physicians. No comprehensive website exists for such evaluations, and as such, many institutions or physicians hide behind the protective mantle of confidentiality.

However, not all is lost, as the momentum towards transparency and freedom of information continues to grow at a much faster pace than before, largely due to the Internet which empowers healthcare consumers regarding available choices when seeking care. Value-based safety and quality data that includes objective safety and quality of care scoring is much needed. It becomes especially valuable when it is linked to cost of care for the consumer. The resulting quality-value matrix will allow for appropriate value-based decisions to be made by the patients when they seek care.

Since consumers must select health plans, medical services, healthcare facilities and physicians, it is imperative that additional safety data be made available to the public. At this time, the selection of a health plan is primarily cost-based and consumers select their physicians by word-of-mouth or location. This is a dangerously inadequate way to make such important decisions.

Some organizations such as The Leapfrog Group have begun to display safety data. Although the Leapfrog Group uses extensive scientific research-based measures developed by the Agency for

Healthcare Quality and Research (AHRQ), the survey data from participating hospitals is self-reported through annual surveys and may be biased. In addition, the survey is voluntary, so it is often completed by hospitals that already are more aggressive in addressing safety concerns.

Although most providers (98%) are aware of incident reporting system, nurses use it more than doctors		
	Nurses	**Doctors**
Have completed an incident report	89.2%	64.6%
Know how to locate/access an incident form	88.3%	43.0%
Know what to do with a completed incident form	81.9%	49.7%

Increasingly, state laws are beginning to mandate the reporting of adverse events and medical errors, especially sentinel events, including hospital acquired infections. Some states are beginning to post this data on public websites, while other states have agreed with hospitals to keep the information confidential and not release it to the public. Nonetheless, the drive is there towards making more of this data available to the public over the next few years.

Ideally, when an error occurs, a national investigative body, independent of the industry itself, should be available to dissect the incident and determine the root causes or sequence of events, much like the National Transportation and Safety Board (NTSB) does when there is an airplane crash. Their investigation and findings would be focused on discovering the truth and taking reparative system wide measures, and not just playing the "blame game" that so often occurs today. Such an organization's final incident evaluation reports, like those of the NTSB, would be made public with a set of recommendations for the industry operators to consider and enforce. Unfortunately, at this time, no such organization exists. There is no federal agency or board to conduct independent investigations of preventable medical errors with non-punitive recommendations and make their findings public.

Assumptions and Communication
Two common denominators were apparent throughout most of the stories in this book:
1. Healthcare professionals making assumptions
2. Healthcare professionals repeatedly failing to listen to patients

Often, physicians and nurses have medical schematics in their heads that quickly lead them to certain conclusions about a patient's diagnosis or condition. These preconceived mechanisms are created through education and experience, and in some cases can save valuable time and wasted effort, but they also can produce tunnel vision and hamper a physician's ability to let in new information.

As stated earlier in this book, doctors may decide on your diagnosis in as little as 18 seconds. Compounding the problem is the very real time constraints placed on how many minutes a doctor can spend with each patient (six minutes on average). This combination leaves no room for the kind of doctor-patient dialogue necessary, given the complexity of healthcare financing today.

Lewis Blackman was viewed as a lazy teenager who did not want to get up and walk instead of as a young man spiraling into a state of shock. It was also assumed that Toradol was safe, when in fact it was harming Lewis and no one thought to check for side effects. Trisha Torrey was perceived as annoying and aggressive, a know-it-all questioning medical science, when in fact she was correct. Ken Simon was immediately diagnosed as suffering a panic attack, although his profile made that highly unlikely, instead of a deadly diagnosis of a dissecting aneurysm. Diana Brookins was assumed to be a drug seeker instead of a young woman in agony due to internal burns and infection. Taylor McCormack was assumed to be safe for a delay in surgery despite major concerns expressed by her parents and critical test values that were ignored. Pregnancy was never considered in Liz Augusta's case because she was taking oral contraceptives.

Each story demonstrates assumptions, all of which resulted in dangerous or deadly outcomes. Every assumption grew out of the experiences of doctors and nurses, who had previously treated people with similar conditions. These experiences blinded them to the possibility that something was very different.

Healthcare professionals need to remove the blinders of assumptions and listen to each and every patient, remembering that each person is an individual, not a disease or surgery or another procedure. Physicians and nurses must be investigators, since nothing is routine in healthcare. Warning signs must be heeded when patients and families speak up. Listening can solve so much!

Every person interviewed for this book was asked the question, "What is the one thing you would tell healthcare professionals?" Without exception, they conveyed the sentiment, "Listen to the patient, and treat them like your own family member." Almost without exception people and their family members spoke up, but no one was hearing what they were trying to say. This phenomenon in hospitals and health systems must stop. The wave of change must quickly and thoroughly wash over today's fractured U.S. healthcare industry.

100 Lives

NUMBER OF LIVES THAT CAN BE SAVED EACH DAY FROM MEDICAL ERRORS IF WE DO THE RIGHT THING

Healthcare consumers must be the ones to drive future changes that will improve healthcare safety for all. It will be a mistake to rely on any government agency, a watchdog group, the U.S. Congress or the healthcare industry itself. Patients must arm themselves with information about their health, medical conditions, treatment options and legal rights. Healthcare consumer will need to stand up and speak up in a more public way by heeding the following:

- Demand data on safety, quality and cost when seeking care
- Become an active participant to drive value-based decisions when seeking care
- Become more informed regarding preventable medical errors from the source of care

- Be an active voice in the healthcare safety reform initiatives being discussed and implemented in your own state and nationally

INFORMATION SOURCES FOR THE EMPOWERED PATIENT

Following are the stories covered in this book and the type of "preventable medical error or adverse event" that occurred:

1. Never Routine: Lewis Blackman—Failure to Rescue
2. Reading Between the Lines: Trisha Torrey—Misdiagnosis (Near Miss)
3. Critically Wounded: Diana Brookins—Bloodstream Infection
4. Picking Up The Pieces: Diane Ford—PCA Pump Failure
5. The Promise: Taylor McCormack—Delay in Treatment
6. Coming Together: Linda Kenney—Medically Induced Trauma
7. One of Their Own: Liz Augusta—Missed Pregnancy (Near Miss)
8. They're Not Listening: Ken Simon—Wrong Diagnosis
9. The Price of Doing Business: Johanna Daly—Surgical Site Infection (SSI)
10. Wrong Turn: Benjamin Houghton—Wrong Side Surgery
11. Three Little Angels: Indiana Babies—Heparin (High-Alert Medication) Overdose

Based on the type of errors, the following are general and error specific informational websites that could one day save your live or the life of someone dear to you. Links to all of these websites and pages are also provided through www.fatalcare.com. Please note that these are all public websites and I am not endorsing any one of these.

GENERAL PATIENT SAFETY & QUALITY OF CARE INFORMATION
The Joint Commission's award-winning patient safety program: Speak Up Initiatives

- http://www.jcipatientsafety.org/14639/
- http://www.jointcommission.org/PatientSafety/SpeakUp/

Facts about Speak Up Initiatives

In March 2002, The Joint Commission, together with the Centers for Medicare and Medicaid Services (CMS), launched a national campaign to urge patients to take a role in preventing healthcare errors by becoming active, involved and informed participants on the healthcare team. The above links and web-pages will give you access to the Speak Up™ program materials - brochures, posters and buttons on a variety of patient safety topics. Speak Up™ was developed to encourage the public to:

- Speak up if you have questions or concerns, and if you don't understand, ask again. It's your body and you have a right to know.
- Pay attention to the care you are receiving. Make sure you're getting the right treatments and medications by the right healthcare professionals. Don't assume anything.
- Educate yourself about your diagnosis, the medical tests you are undergoing, and your treatment plan.
- Ask a trusted family member or friend to be your advocate.
- Know what medications you take and why you take them. Medication errors are the most common healthcare mistakes.
- Use a hospital, clinic, surgery center, or other type of healthcare organization that has undergone a rigorous on-site evaluation against established state-of-the-art quality and safety standards, such as that provided by The Joint Commission.
- Participate in all decisions about your treatment. You are the center of the healthcare team.

Reference: http://www.jointcommission.org/PatientSafety/
SpeakUp/about_speakup.htm

Patient Safety Advocacy Support Groups/Diagnosis Errors
Trisha Torrey's Websites:
- www.diagKNOWsis.org This website has the resources and links
  to empower you with the tools you need to make tough medical
  decisions, especially when it comes to life threatening diagnoses.

- www.EveryPatientsAdvocate.com
  Every Patient's Advocate™ has one important purpose: to help
  patients learn everything they can about advocating for good
  health and medical care for themselves or their loved ones.

  The information on this site is presented for patients, by
  a former patient, from a patient's point of view. . . . to help
  patients become good healthcare consumers by providing
  them with the tools they need to do so. As a part of the
  DiagKNOWsis family of websites, Every Patient's Advocate
  provides columns and podcasts which can be shared through
  publication in consumer-read newspapers, magazines, e-zines or
  through audio media.

AHRQ Patient Safety Network (PSNet)
- http://psnet.ahrq.gov/index.aspx

The above link is to the AHRQ Patient Safety Network (PSNet)
website. This is a new national web-based resource featuring the latest
news and essential resources on patient safety. The site offers weekly
updates of patient safety literature, news, tools, and meetings ("What's
New"), and a vast set of carefully annotated links to important
research and other information on patient safety ("The Collection").
Supported by a robust patient safety taxonomy and web architecture,
AHRQ PSNet provides powerful searching and browsing capability,
as well as the ability for diverse users to customize the site around

their interests (My PSNet). It also is tightly coupled with AHRQ WebM&M, the popular monthly journal that features user-submitted cases of medical errors, expert commentaries, and perspectives on patient safety.

AHRQ PSNet and AHRQ WebM&M are both funded by the Agency for Healthcare Research and Quality and edited by a team at the University of California, San Francisco, with the technical support of Silverchair
    • AHRQ Web M&M can be accessed via http://webmm.ahrq.gov
    The AHRQ Morbidity and Mortality Rounds on the Web is the online journal and forum on patient safety and healthcare quality. This site features expert analysis of medical errors reported anonymously by our readers, interactive learning modules on patient safety ("Spotlight Cases"), Perspectives on Safety, and forums for online discussion. CME and CEU credit are available.
    AHRQ WebM&M is funded by the Agency for Healthcare Research and Quality, edited by a team at the University of California San Francisco, with the technical support of Silverchair. An Editorial Board and Advisory Panel, comprised of experts in patient safety, healthcare quality, and clinical disciplines, guide the editorial team.
    AHRQ WebM&M was launched in February 2003. This site is dedicated to the memory of the late AHRQ Director Dr. John Eisenberg, who originally envisioned it.
    • Patient Safety Terms Glossary can be accessed via http://psnet
     .ahrq.gov/glossary.aspx#F

The Joint Commission's Quality Check program
    • This program can be accessed via www.qualitycheck.org

Quality Check—www.qualitycheck.org—is a comprehensive guide to healthcare organizations in the United States. Visitors can search by city and state, or by name and zip code (up to 250 miles).
    The Joint Commission has had a longstanding commitment to providing meaningful information about the comparative performance of accredited organizations to the public. In 1994, the

Joint Commission first published organization-specific Performance Reports. In 1996, Quality Check®, a directory of Joint Commission accredited organizations and performance reports, became available on the website. In 2004, Quality Reports replaced Performance Reports, although historical Performance Reports are still available.

Quality Reports on Healthcare Organizations from the Quality Check Website

Quality Reports feature a user-friendly format with checks, pluses and minuses to help the general public compare healthcare organization performance in a number of key areas. While Quality Check displays demographic and service information for organizations not accredited by the Joint Commission on the Quality Check Search Results page, Quality Reports are only available for organizations that are accredited by the Joint Commission. Quality Reports provide information about a healthcare organization's:

- Joint Commission accreditation decision and the effective dates of the accreditation award. For Provisional, Conditional, and Preliminary Denial of Accreditation decisions, the reports will list the standards cited for Requirements for Improvement.
- Programs accredited by the Joint Commission, and programs or services accredited by other accrediting bodies.
- Compliance with the Joint Commission's National Patient Safety Goals, as applicable to the organization.
- Performance on National Quality Improvement Goals (hospitals only). These goals allow hospitals to report on key quality of care indicators in up to five treatment areas: heart attack, heart failure, community acquired pneumonia, pregnancy and related conditions, and surgical care improvement project for infection prevention. This performance data is updated quarterly. As more measures are approved and endorsed by the National Quality Forum, the Joint Commission will explore ways to incorporate that data in Quality Reports.
- Special quality awards, including recognition such as Disease-Specific Care Certification, Ernest A. Codman Award, Eisenberg Patient Safety Award, Franklin Award, and Magnet

status (awarded by the American Nurses Credentialing Center), Medal of Honor for Organ Donation and others approved by the Joint Commission Board of Commissioners.

New in 2007 on the Quality Check Program

- As of October 1, the Joint Commission's Quality Check website includes organizations that are not accredited by the Joint Commission as well as Joint Commission accredited organizations. Joint Commission accredited organizations are easily identified by the Joint Commission's Gold Seal of Approval™.
- Organizations not accredited by the Joint Commission can request to be added to Quality Check by accessing www.qualitycheck.org/qcdirectory.
- The search function has been expanded so that users can find organizations by type of service provided within a geographic area. Once a service and area have been selected, the healthcare organizations displayed can be filtered by type of provider, setting of care or patient population. Some of the pre-defined services that can be selected for search are cardiac care, developmental disabilities, dialysis, home medical equipment, neurology, occupational health and optometry.
- The search results page now includes a cleaner display for readability, a special quality awards display, a link to view all services provided at the healthcare organization's sites, and links to directions and websites for the healthcare organization, when available.

New in 2008 on the Quality Check Program

- Quality Reports for organizations that have pursued disease-specific care certification. The initial reports will include listings of certifications by site and performance against the National Patient Safety Goals.

Sentinel Event Alerts
- The Joint Commission posts alerts on serious patient safety events and mishaps. These can be accessed from the following site:

  http://www.jointcommission.org/SentinelEvents/ SentinelEventAlert/

The Center for Medicare and Medicaid Services (CMS) Hospital Compare Program

The Hospital Compare website was created through the efforts of the Centers for Medicare & Medicaid Services (CMS), an agency of the U.S. Department of Health and Human Services (DHHS), along with the Hospital Quality Alliance (HQA). The HQA is a public-private collaboration established to promote reporting on hospital quality of care. The HQA consists of organizations that represent consumers, hospitals, doctors, nurses, employers, accrediting organizations, and federal agencies. The information on the Hospital Compare website can be accessed via the URL below and used by any adult needing hospital care:

www.hospitalcompare.hhs.gov/

Hospital Compare displays rates for Process of Care measures that show how often hospitals provide some of the care that is recommended for patients being treated for a heart attack, heart failure or pneumonia, and patients having surgery. Hospitals voluntarily submit data from their medical records about the treatments their adult patients receive for these conditions, including patients with Medicare and those who do not have Medicare.

This information can help you, your healthcare provider, family, and friends to compare the quality of care provided in the hospitals where you receive care. This type of quality of care information not only helps you make good decisions about your healthcare, but also encourages hospitals to improve the quality of healthcare they provide.

Report a Complaint About a Healthcare Organization
If you have a complaint about the quality of care at a Joint
Commission-accredited healthcare organization, then the Joint
Commission (TJC) wants to know about it. You can submit your
complaint online or send it by mail, fax, or e-mail. To access the
Joint Commission complaint reporting website go to: http://www.
jointcommission
.org/GeneralPublic/Complaint/

MEDICATION ERRORS

Medication errors are one of the most frequently occurring types of
preventable adverse event that affects patients within our healthcare
system. The National Coordinating Council for Medication Error
Reporting and Prevention (NCC-MERP) defines a medication error
as:

Any preventable event that may cause or lead to inappropriate
medication use or patient harm while the medication is in the control
of the healthcare professional, patient, or consumer. Such events may
be related to professional practice, healthcare products, procedures,
and systems, including prescribing; order communication; product
labeling, packaging, and nomenclature; compounding; dispensing;
distribution; administration; education; monitoring; and use.

The American Hospital Association (AHA) lists the following as
some common types of medication errors:

- incomplete patient information (not knowing about patients'
  allergies, other medicines they are taking, previous diagnoses,
  and lab results, for example);
- unavailable drug information (such as lack of up-to-date
  warnings);
- miscommunication of drug orders, which can involve poor
  handwriting, confusion between drugs with similar names,
  misuse of zeroes and decimal points, confusion of metric and
  other dosing units, and inappropriate abbreviations;
- lack of appropriate labeling as a drug is prepared and repackaged
  into smaller units; and

- Environmental factors, such as lighting, heat, noise, and interruptions, which can distract health professionals from their medical tasks.

The following websites and organizations have useful information and services that can aid you in understanding medication errors better:

Institute for Safe Medication Practices
Phone: (215) 947-7797
Fax: (215) 914-1492
http://www.ismp.org/default.asp

The Institute for Safe Medication Practices (ISMP), based in suburban Philadelphia, is the nation's only 501c (3) nonprofit organization devoted entirely to medication error prevention and safe medication use. ISMP represents over 30 years of experience in helping healthcare practitioners keep patients safe, and continues to lead efforts to improve the medication use process. The organization is known and respected worldwide as the premier resource for impartial, timely, and accurate medication safety information.

The Institute has a long history of achievements. Its medication error prevention efforts began in 1975 with a groundbreaking and continuing column in *Hospital Pharmacy* that increases understanding and educates healthcare professionals and others about medication error prevention. In 2004, the Institute celebrated the 10th anniversary of its official incorporation as a nonprofit organization.

Today, a continuously expanding core of knowledge in medication safety fuels the Institute's highly effective initiatives to improve the medication use process. These initiatives, which are built upon a non-punitive approach and system-based solutions, fall into five key areas: knowledge, analysis, education, cooperation, and communication.

Food and Drug Administration (FDA)

FDA receives medication error reports on marketed human drugs (including prescription drugs, generic drugs, and over-the-counter drugs) and non-vaccine biological products and devices.

In 1992, the FDA began monitoring medication error reports that are forwarded to FDA from the United States Pharmacopeia (USP) and the Institute for Safe Medication Practices (ISMP). The Agency also reviews MedWatch reports for possible medication errors. Currently, medication errors are reported to the FDA as manufacturer reports (adverse events resulting in serious injury and for which a medication error may be a component), direct contact reports (MedWatch), or reports from USP or ISMP.

- FDA receives medication error reports on marketed human drugs (including prescription drugs, generic drugs, and over-the-counter drugs) and non-vaccine biological products and devices. The following link will take you to a FDA web-page that provides very useful links to information on medication errors:

  http://www.fda.gov/cder/drug/MedErrors/default.htm

- Medications and Older People: The Food and Drug Administration is working to make drugs safer for older people, who consume a large share of the nation's medications. People over age 65 buy 30 percent of all prescription drugs and 40 percent of all OTC drugs. The following FDA web-page is for information on medication errors associated with the older adult:

  http://www.fda.gov/FDAC/features/1997/697_old.html

American Society of Health-System Pharmacists (ASHP)
The American Society of Health-System Pharmacists (ASHP) is the 30,000-member national professional association comprised of pharmacists who work with doctors and other health professionals in:
- Hospitals,
- Ambulatory care clinics, and
- Long-term care and home care facilities

ASHP's mission is to support pharmacists in helping people use medications safely and effectively.
- Medications Database: The drug information in this searchable database is based on *ASHP's Medication Teaching Manual: The*

Guide to Patient Drug Information, a publication developed for use in patient-education programs conducted by health-care professionals. The database, which features more than 900 name-brand and generic medicines, is designed to supplement information provided by your physician and the pharmacist who dispenses your prescriptions. Always consult with your pharmacist or physician directly if you have questions about the medicines you take.

The following website will provide you with drug information from a searchable database, based on *ASHP's Medication Teaching Manual: The Guide to Patient Drug Information*, a publication developed for use in patient-education programs conducted by health-care professionals. The database, which features more than 900 name-brand and generic medicines, is designed to supplement information provided by your physician and the pharmacist who dispenses your prescriptions:

http://www.safemedication.com/About/medMaster.cfm

Medication Safety Guide from the Agency for Healthcare Research and Quality (AHRQ)

You can learn more about how to take medicines safely by reading this guide. It answers common questions about getting and taking medicines and has many handy forms that will help you keep track of information. Keep this guide with your medicines in case you have any questions, concerns, or worries.

http://www.ahrq.gov/consumer/safemeds/safemeds.htm

This guide was developed by the Agency for Healthcare Research and Quality (AHRQ) and the National Council on Patient Information and Education (NCPIE).

HOSPITAL ACQUIRED INFECTIONS
Consumer Website to Stop Hospital Infections
The following URL is an excellent website with very good links to

several resources on hospital infections:

http://www.consumersunion.org/campaigns/
stophospitalinfections/learn.html

The site is managed by the Consumers Union (CU), which is an expert, independent, nonprofit organization. The CU's mission is to work for a fair, just, and safe marketplace for all consumers. CU publishes *Consumer Reports* and ConsumerReports.org in addition to two newsletters, *Consumer Reports on Health* and *Consumer Reports Money Adviser* with combined subscriptions of more than 7 million people. Consumers Union also has more than 500,000 online activists who help work to change legislation and the marketplace in favor of the consumer interest and several public education Web sites. Since its founding in 1936, Consumers Union has never taken any advertising or freebies of any kind.

Centers for Disease Control
The Centers for Disease Control has several programs and resources to address healthcare acquired infections and is an excellent resource for consumers. Following are a few links from the CDC that are specific to preventable infections:

- The National Nosocomial Infections Surveillance (NNIS) system has now been replaced by the National Healthcare Safety Network [NHSN]). The NNIS was started initially to monitor the incidence of healthcare-associated (nosocomial) infections (HAIs) and their associated risk factors and pathogens. The NHSN has a broader objective.
  - http://www.cdc.gov/ncidod/dhqp/nnis.html
- CDC pages on healthcare-acquired infections and community-acquired infections can be accessed via the following URL:
  - http://www.cdc.gov/ncidod/dhqp/healthDis.html

FAILURE TO RESCUE (FTR)
As defined by AHRQ, "Failure to rescue" is shorthand for failure to rescue (i.e., prevent a clinically important deterioration, such as death

or permanent disability) from a complication of an underlying illness (e.g., cardiac arrest in a patient with acute myocardial infarction) or a complication of medical care (e.g., major hemorrhage after thrombolysis for acute myocardial infarction). Monitoring failure to rescue provides a measure of the degree by which providers respond to adverse occurrences (e.g., hospital-acquired infections, cardiac arrest or shock).

WRONG DIAGNOSIS OR MISDIAGNOSIS
WrongDiagnosis.com (http://www.wrongdiagnosis.com/)
This is one of the world's leading providers of online medical health information. The site is an independent, objective source of factual, mainstream health information for both consumers and health professionals.

WrongDiagnosis.com provides a free health-information service to help people understand their health better, offering crucial and factual health information that is otherwise difficult to find. The objective of the site is to encourage consumers to be informed and interested in managing their health, and to know what questions to ask their doctors to help ensure they are getting the best healthcare possible.

Cureresearch.com (http://www.cureresearch.com/intro/overview.htm)
This is a good website for diagnosis and treatment information. This web site is managed by Adviware Pty Ltd, an independent technology company that is not affiliated with any medical or drug organization. This means the factual, mainstream information presented is unbiased.

MEDICALLY INDUCED TRAUMA
Medically Induced Trauma Support Services (MITSS) (http://www .mitss.org/)

Medically Induced Trauma Support Services (MITSS), Inc. is a non-profit organization founded in June of 2002 whose mission is *"To Support Healing and Restore Hope"* to patients, families, and clinicians who have been affected by an adverse medical event.

Medically induced trauma is an unexpected outcome that occurs during medical and/or surgical care that affects the emotional well being of the patient, family member, or clinician. MITSS achieves its mission by:

- Creating Awareness and Education—Since 2002, MITSS has been educating the healthcare community on the uniqueness of medical trauma, the broad scope of its impact, and the crucial need for support services through participation in forums, local and national conferences, and through the media.
- Direct Support Services to Patients, Families, and Clinicians—MITSS provides educational support groups for patients and their families who have been affected by medical error or unanticipated outcomes led by a clinical psychologist. MITSS also provides support groups for nursing professionals finding themselves at the "sharp end" of an adverse medical event.
- Advocacy for Action— "We encourage and consult with healthcare institutions in developing infrastructures for clinician peer support systems. We also assist in developing a referral process to the MITSS program for patients and families."

WRONG-SIDE, SITE, PROCEDURE AND PERSON SURGERY

The Joint Commission (TJC) Universal Protocol for preventing such mishaps

In July 2003, the Joint Commission Board of Commissioners approved the Universal Protocol for Preventing Wrong Site, Wrong Procedure and Wrong Person Surgery™. The Universal Protocol was created to address the continuing occurrence of these tragic medical errors in Joint Commission accredited organizations. The Universal Protocol became effective July 1, 2004 for all accredited hospitals, ambulatory care and office-based surgery facilities. The Universal

Protocol drew upon, and expanded and integrated, a series of requirements under the Joint Commission's 2003 and 2004 National Patient Safety Goals. It is applicable to all operative and other invasive procedures. The principal components of the Universal Protocol include: 1) the pre-operative verification process; 2) marking of the operative site; 3) taking a 'time-out' immediately before starting the procedure; and 4) adaptation of the requirements to non-operating room settings, including bedside procedures. The protocol is endorsed by 51 professional healthcare associations and organizations.

Wrong site, wrong procedure and wrong person surgeries are sentinel events (an unexpected occurrence involving death or serious physical or psychological injury) that are tracked through the Joint Commission sentinel event database. The Joint Commission has issued two *Sentinel Event Alert* newsletters on the subject of wrong site surgery; the first was published August 28, 1998, and the follow-up issue was published December 5, 2001. In response to continuing reports of wrong site, wrong procedure and wrong person surgery, Joint Commission leadership agreed that it was necessary to get key organizations involved in efforts to prevent wrong site, wrong procedure and wrong person surgery. The universal protocol can be accessed from:

- http://www.jointcommission.org/PatientSafety/Universal Protocol/wss_tips.htm

REFERENCES

CHAPTER 1— NEVER ROUTINE

1. Monk, J. (2002, June 16). Lewis Blackman. *The State*: SPECIAL REPORT, pp. A1, A8-9. Retrieved on February 18, 2007 from http://www.lewis blackman.net/

2. Monk, J. (2007, January 28). Hospitals launching patient safety initiatives. New measures are aimed at making more information available to the public. *The State*. Retrieved on February 18, 2007 from http://www.thestate.com/mld/thestate/16562686.htm

3. Drachman, A., Ellis, R., Turner, D. (2005, August). Lewis Blackman Patient Safety Act, South Carolina SC Code Ann.§44-7-3410 *et seq.* Retrieved February 20, 2007 from http://www.musc.edu/medcenter/trainingToolbox/ClinEd/LewBlkm_files/frame.htm

4. Wikipedia, (2007). *Residency.* Retrieved February 22, 2007 from http://en.wikipedia.org/wiki/Residency_(medicine)

5. Chassim, M.R., & Becher, E.C. (2002, June 4). The wrong patient. *Annals of Internal Medicine*, 136(11), 826-833. University Health System Consortium. Rapid Response Teams. Retrieved February 24, 2007 from http://public.uhc.edu/uhcmail/ihi/rrt.htm

6. The Joint Commission. (2007). Hospital/Critical Access Hospital National Patient Safety Goals. Retrieved February 24, 2007 from http://www.jointcommission.org/PatientSafety/NationalPatientSafetyGoals/07_hap_cah_npsgs.htm

7. Wikipedia. (2007). *Attending Physician.* Retrieved February 24, 2007 from http://en.wikipedia.org/wiki/Attending_physician

8. Lieberman, T. (2004, November).Your health, fatal mistakes. *AARP.* Retrieved February 25, 2007 from http://www.aarp.org/bulletin/yourhealth/a2004-10-27-fatal_mistakes.html

9. Silber JH, Williams SV, Krakauer H, Schwartz JS. Hospital and patient characteristics associated with death after surgery. A study of adverse occurrence and failure to rescue. Med Care. 1992;30:615-629.

10. Aiken LH, Clarke SP, Sloane DM, Sochalski J, Silber JH. Hospital nurse staffing and patient mortality, nurse burnout, and job dissatisfaction. JAMA. 2002;288:1987-1993.

11. Needleman J, Buerhaus P, Mattke S, Stewart M, Zelevinsky K. Nurse-staffing levels and the quality of care in hospitals. N Engl J Med. 2002;346:1715-1722.

12. Aiken LH, Clarke SP, Cheung RB, Sloane DM, Silber JH. Educational levels of hospital nurses and surgical patient mortality. JAMA. 2003;290:1617-1623.

13. McDonald KM, Romano PS, Geppert J, et al. Measures of Patient Safety Based on Hospital Administrative Data—The Patient Safety Indicators. Rockville, MD: Agency for Healthcare Research and Quality; 2002. AHRQ Publication No. 02-0038. Available at: http://www.ahrq.gov/clinic/evrptfiles .htm#psi.

CHAPTER 2—READING - BETWEEN THE LINES

1. Kohn, L.T, Corrigan, J.M. & Donaldson, M.S. (Eds.). (1999). *To err is human: building a safer health system.* Institute of Medicine. Washington, D.C.: National Academy Press.

2. Berntsen, K.J. (2004). *The patient's guide to preventing medical errors.* Westport, CT: Praeger Publishing Group.

3. Jelic, S. (2005, November, 26). Second opinions - why it's important to get a second opinion. About.com. Retrieved May 16, 2007 from http://lung diseases.about.com/od/lungcancer/a/secondopinions.htm

4. O'Niel, P. (rev). (2006, September 1). Breast Cancer, Seeking a Second Doctor's Opinion. WebMD. Retrieved May 14, 2007. From http://www. webmd.com/breast-cancer/guide/seeking-second-opinion.

5. National Cancer Institute. (2007). Interpreting Laboratory Test Results, Fact Sheet. Retrieved November 24, 2007 from http://www.cancer.gov/cancer

topics/factsheet/Detection/laboratory-tests
6. Leonhardt, D. (2006, February, 22).Why doctors so often get it wrong. *The New York Times: Business*. Retrieved May 15, 2007 from http://www.isabel healthcare.com/info/newyorktime.html

CHAPTER 3—CRITICALLY WOUNDED

1. National Digestive Disease Information Clearing House. (2004, November 29). ERCP. Retrieved March 24, 2007 from http://digestive.niddk.nih.gov/ddiseases/pubs/ercp/index.htm
2. Sherertz, R.J., Ely, E.W., Westbrook, D.M., et al. (2000). Education of physicians-in-training can decrease the risk for vascular catheter infection. *Ann Intern Med*,132:641-8.
3. Stephens, S.S., Lauze, D., Bellush, M.J. (2005, October 14). Reduction in central line associated bloodstream infections among patients in intensive care units, Pennsylvania, April 2001-March 2005. Centers for Disease Control, 54(40);1013-1016. Retrieved March 25, 2007 from http://www.cdc.gov/mmwr/preview/mmwrhtml/mm5440a2.htm
4. Pearson M.L. (1996). Guideline for prevention of intravascular device-related infections. Part I. Intravascular device-related infections: an overview. The Hospital Infection Control Practices Advisory Committee. *American Journal of Infect Control*, 24:262-77.

CHAPTER 4—PICKING UP THE PIECES

1. Institute for Safe Medication Practices. (2002, May, 29). *Medication Safety Alert, More on avoiding opiate toxicity with PCA by proxy*. Retrieved April 14, 2007 from http://www.ismp.org/newsletters/acutecare/articles/20020529.asp
2. Institute for Safe Medication Practices. (2003, July 28). *Pain control in hospitals using PCA pumps, must be made safer*. Retrieved April 14, 2007 from http://www.ismp.org/pressroom/PR20030728.pdf
3. Drugs@FDA. Label and approval history. *Narcan*. Retrieved April 14, 2007 from http://www.accessdata.fda.gov/scripts/cder/drugsatfda/index.cfm?fuseaction=Search.Label_ApprovalHistory#apphist
4. Reves, J. G. (2003, Spring). Anesthesia Patient Safety Foundation Newsletter.

Smart pump technology reduces errors. Retrieved April 15, 2007 from http://www.apsf.org/resource_center/newsletter/2003/spring/smartpump.htm

5. Ford, D. An essay on patient safety. *Colorado Patient Safety Coalition.* Retrieved on April 15, 2007 from http://www.coloradopatientsafety.org/danfordessay.htm

CHAPTER 5—THE PROMISE

1. Kuperman, G. J., Boyle, D., Jha., et al. (1998, February 5). How promptly are inpatients treated for critical laboratory results? *JAMIA*, 112-119. Retrieved November 22, 2007 from http://www.pubmedcentral.nih.gov/articlerender.fcgi?artid=61280

2. Sood, S., Canady, A.I., Ham, S.D. (2000). Evaluation of shunt malfunctions using shunt site reservoir. *Pediatric Neurosurgery*, 32(4). Retrieved April2, 2007 from http://content.karger.com/ProdukteDB/produkte.asp?Aktion =ShowFulltext&ProduktNr=224273&Ausgabe=226508&ArtikelNr=28931

3. Mayo Clinic. (2007, September 12). Tools for a healthier live. Hydrocephalus. Retrieved September 30, 2007 from http://www.mayoclinic.com/health/hydrocephalus/DS00393

4. Taylor McCormack Memorial. (2007). http://memorial2taylor.com/index.html

5. Agency for Healthcare Research and Quality. (2004, June 7). Children in hospitals frequently experience medical injuries - Press Release. Retrieved November 24, 2007 from http://www.ahrq.gov/news/press/pr2004/chhosppr .htm

6. Barnard, A. (2003, September 20). Nurse disputes events in death at children's. *Boston Globe*. Retrieved on March 10, 2007 from http://www .boston.com/news/local/articles/2003/09/20/nurse_disputes_events_in_ death_at_childrens/

CHAPTER 6—COMING TOGETHER

1. Wikipedia. (2007). Bupivacaine. Retrieved April 29, 2007 from http://en.wikipedia.org/wiki/Bupivacaine

2. Medically Induced Trauma Support Services (MITSS). (2007). Mission, purpose and vision. Retrieved April 29, 2007 from http://www.mitss.org/aboutus_home.html

3. Anesthesia Patient Safety Foundation. (2007). Mission statement and history. Retrieved April 28, 2007 from http://www.apsf.org/about/

4. Berntsen, K.J. (2004). *The patient's guide to preventing medical errors*. Westport, CT: Praeger Publishing Group.

5. Eichhorn, J. H. (2005). Patient perspectives personalize patient safety. *Anesthesia Patient Safety Foundation workshop*. Retrieved April 28, 2007 from http://www.apsf.org/resource_center/newsletter/2006/winter/01perspective.htm

CHAPTER 7—ONE OF THEIR OWN

1. Food and Drug Administration. (2007). Pregnancy Categories of Drug Safety.

2. Toppenberg, K. S., Hill, A. D., Miller, D. P. (1999, April 1). Safety of radiographic imaging during pregnancy. *American Family Physician*. Retrieved May 12, 2007 from http://www.aafp.org/afp/990401ap/1813.html

3. Hall E.J. (1991). Scientific view of low-level radiation risks. Radiographics, 11:509-18.

4. Food and Drug Administration. (2001, May 11). CDRM Consumer information, X-rays, pregnancy and you. *HHS Publication* No., 94-8087. Retrieved May 12, 2007 from http://www.fda.gov/cdrh/consumer/xraypreg.html

5. Web MD. (2007). Magnetic resonance angiogram (MRA). *Heart Disease Health Center*. Retrieved May 13, 2007 from http://www.webmd.com/heart-disease/Magnetic-Resonance-Angiogram-MRA

6. Sandler, T.W. (2004). Lippincott Williams &Wilkins. Langman's Medical Embryology. 9th Edition. Retrieved May 13, 2007 from http://books.google.com/books?id=VaRMUFUdRSsC&printsec=frontcover&dq=pregnant+woman+birth+defects+Nagasaki+and+Hiroshima,#PPR9,M1

7 Begelman, S.M. (2004, August 2). What is Fibromuscular Dysplasia (FMD)? *Fibromuscular Dysplasia Society of America Inc*. Retrieved May 20, 2007 from http://www.fmdsa.org/about_fmd.html

CHAPTER 8—THEY'RE NOT LISTENING

1. Cleveland Clinic. (2006). Surgery for thoracic aortic aneurysm. *Heart & Vascular Institute*. Retrieved May 25, 2007 from http://www.clevelandclinic

.org/heartcenter/pub/guide/disease/aorta_marfan/surgerythoracicaneurysm
.htm?id=cff00046&engine=adwords&keyword=aortic+aneurysm&WT
.srch=1&WT.mc&?id=cff00046&gclid=CIKP-dvJqYwCFQNYYQodMx
GhMQ

2. Mayoclinic.com. (2007). Tools for healthier living. Heart Disease. Aortic
Aneurysm. Retrieved May 25, 2007 from http://www.mayoclinic.com/health/
aortic-aneurysm/DS00017

3. Live and learn. (2007). Aneurysm Aortic. *American Heart Association*.
Retrieved May 27, 2007 from http://www.americanheart.org/presenter
.jhtml?identifier=4455

4. Wikipedia. (2007).Aorta Aneurysm. Retrieved May 27, 2007 from http://
en.wikipedia.org/wiki/Aortic_aneurism

5. Kellermann, A. L. (2006, September 28). Crisis in the emergency
department, perspective *New England Journal of Medicine*, 355:1300-1303.
Retrieved May 27, 2007 from http://content.nejm.org/cgi/content/
full/355/13/1300

6. The National Academies Press, (2006, April). *Hospital based emergency care:
at the breaking point*. Retrieved May 27, 2007 from http://www.iom
.edu/?id=35025

7. ABC's Good Morning America. (2006, September 17). Illinois woman's
ER wait death ruled homicide. Long ER waits plague nation's hospitals.
Retrieved May 24, 2007 from http://abcnews.go.com/GMA/Health/
story?id=2454685&page=1

8. Ornstein, C. (2007, June 2). Tale of the last 90 minutes of a woman's life. *Los
Angles Times*.

9. Salyer, S.A. (2006, August 6). Lesson in healing, case becomes an example at
providence. *The HeraldNet*. Retricved May 25, 2007 from http://www.herald
net.com/stories/06/08/06/100loc_a1healing001.cfm

CHAPTER 9—THE PRICE OF DOING BUSINESS

1. Centers for Disease Control and Prevention, (1994). National Center
for Health Statistics Vital and Health Statistics, Detailed diagnoses and
procedures national hospital discharge survey: 127. Hyattsville, MD.
Department of Health and Human Services.

2. Berntsen, K.J. (2004). The patient's guide to preventing medical errors.

Westport, CT: Praeger Publishing Group.

3. Nichols, R.L. (2001, March-April). Preventing surgical site infections: A surgeon's perspective. Emerging Infectious Diseases. Centers for Disease Control. Retrieved May 28, 2007 from http://www.cdc.gov/ncidod/eid/vol7no2/nichols.htm

4. Institute of Healthcare Improvement. (2007). Surgical site infections. case for improvement. Retrieved May 28, 2007 from http://www.ihi.org/ihi/Topics/PatientSafety/SurgicalSiteInfections/SurgicalSiteInfectionsCaseForImprovement

5. Horan, T.C., et al, (1992). Definition of nosocomial infections. Centers of Disease Control: 606-08.

6. Gottrup, F., Helling, A., Hollander, D. (2005, May 2). World wide wounds. An overview of surgical site infections, etiology, incidents and risk factors. Retrieved June 2, 2007 from http://www.worldwidewounds.com/2005/september/Gottrup/Surgical-Site-Infections-Overview.html

CHAPTER 10—WRONG TURN

1. Engel, M. (2007, April 5). Tribune Newspapers: *Los Angeles Times.*

2. Kwaan M.R., Studdert D.M., Zinner M.J., Gawande A.A. (2006). Incidence, patterns, and prevention of wrong-site surgery. *Arch Surg*:141:353-358.

3. DiJoseph, S. (2006 April 1). California Hospital Announces New Rules after Opening Wrong Side of Child's Skull during Brain Surgery. *News Inferno.com*,. Retrieved May 5, 2007 from http://www.newsinferno.com/archives/1038

4. Meinberg, E. G., Stern, P. J. (2003). Incidence of Wrong-Site Surgery Among Hand Surgeons. *The Journal of Bone and Joint Surgery:* 85:193–197. Retrieved May 5, 2007 from http://www.ejbjs.org/cgi/content/abstract/85/2/193

CHAPTER 11—THREE LITTLE ANGELS

1. Aspden, P., Wolcott, J., Bootman, J.L., Cronenwett, L.R. (Eds.). (2006). *Preventing medication errors.* Quality Chasm Series. Institute of Medicine. Washington, D.C.: National Academy Press.

2. Institute for Safe Medication Practices. (1999, June 16). Medication Alert: *Survey of automated dispensing shows need for practice improvements and safer system design.* Retrieved on January 25, 2007 from http://www.ismp.org/Newsletters/acutecare/articles/19990616.asp

3. McGrath, J.M. Neonatal Intensive Care Units. *Neonatal Intensive Care Forum.* Retrieved January 20, 2007 from http://www.deathreference.com/Me-Nu/Neonatal-Intensive-Care-Unit.html

4. Berntsen, K.J. (2004). *The patient's guide to preventing medical errors.* Westport, CT: Praeger Publishing Group.

5. Heparin error background. (2006, September 20). Retrieved January 28, 2007 from http://www.medicine.iu.edu/documents/Scope%20Content/Heparin%20error%20backgrounder.pdf

6. Uhi, D., Eskew, J., Shahriari, V., Ward, D. (2007). *Lessons Learned: The Aftermath of the Heparin Event at Methodist Hospital.* Indianapolis..

7. Kaushal R., Bates D.W., Landrigan C., et al. (2001). Medication errors and adverse events in pediatric inpatients. JAMA, 286.2114020.

8. USP. Top 50 drugs products associated with medication errors. (2003). Retrieved January 29, 2007 from http://www.usp.org/patientSafety/resources/top50DrugErrors.html

9. Clarian Newsroom. (2006, September, 17). *Heparin incident at Methodist Hospital's Newborn Intensive Care Unit.* Retrieved February 2, 2007 from http://www.clarian.org/portal/patients/news?clarianContentID=/health/announcements/20060918_odle.xml

10. Tiernon, A.M. (2007, February, 12). WTHR Eyewitness News. Infant death leads to procedural changes at Methodist. Retrieved February 3, 2007 from http://www.wthr.com/Global/story.asp?S=5424070

11. Kusmer, K. (2006, September 20). WHAS11. *3rd premature infant dies of overdose at Indianapolis hospital.* Retrieved February 3, 2007 from http://www.whas11.com/sharedcontent/APStories/stories/D8K8O2G80.html

12. Bates, D.W., Cullen, D.J., Lard, M.N., et al. (1995). Incidence of adverse drug events and potential adverse drug events: Implications and prevention. *JAMA*; 274: 29-34.

13. Cohen, M. (2004, January). *A vial situation. Heparin Overdose.* Retrieved January 28, 2007 from http://findarticles.com/p/articles/mi_qa3689/is_200401/ai_n9398213